# $\mathscr{B}$ASIC INFECTION CONTROL
## FOR
## HEALTH CARE PROVIDERS

8/04

D1159279

This book is dedicated to the love of my life—
my bride, Trisha.

# Basic Infection Control
# for
# Health Care Providers

▼ ▼ ▼ ▼ ▼ ▼ ▼

### Mike Kennamer, MPA, EMT-P

Director
Department of Emergency Medical Services
Northeast Alabama Community College
Rainsville, Alabama

**DELMAR**

**THOMSON LEARNING**   Australia   Canada   Mexico   Singapore   Spain   United Kingdom   United States

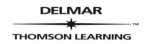

# Basic Infection Control for Health Care Providers

Mike Kennamer

**Health Care Publishing Director:**
William Brottmiller

**Executive Editor:**
Cathy L. Esperti

**Acquisitions Editor:**
Maureen Muncaster

**Editorial Assistant:**
Jill Korznat

**Executive Marketing Manager:**
Dawn F. Gerrain

**Production Editor:**
James Zayicek

COPYRIGHT © 2002 by Delmar, a division of Thomson Learning, Inc. Thomson Learning ™ is a trademark used herein under license.

Printed in the United States of America
2 3 4 5 XXX 06 05 04

For more information contact Delmar,
3 Columbia Circle, PO Box 15015,
Albany, NY 12212-5015

Or find us on the World Wide Web at
http://www.delmar.com

ALL RIGHTS RESERVED. No part of this work covered by the copyright hereon may be reproduced or used in any form or by any means—graphic, electronic, or mechanical, including photocopying, recording, taping, Web distribution, or information storage and retrieval systems—without written permission of the publisher.

For permission to use material from this text or product, contact us by
Tel   (800) 730-2214
Fax   (800) 730-2215
www.thomsonrights.com

Library of Congress Cataloging-in-Publication Data
Kennamer, Mike.
  Basic infection control for health care providers / Mike Kennamer.
    p. cm.
  Includes index.
  ISBN 0-7668-2678-3
    1. Nosocomial infections—Prevention. 2. Medical personnel—Health and hygiene. 3. Health facilities—Sanitation. I. Title.

RA969 .K46 200l
614.4'4—dc21                                    2001047035

## NOTICE TO THE READER

Publisher does not warrant or guarantee any of the products described herein or perform any independent analysis in connection with any of the product information contained herein. Publisher does not assume, and expressly disclaims, any obligation to obtain and include information other than that provided to it by the manufacturer.

The reader is expressly warned to consider and adopt all safety precautions that might be indicated by the activities herein and to avoid all potential hazards. By following the instructions contained herein, the reader willingly assumes all risks in connection with such instructions.

The Publisher makes no representation or warranties of any kind, including but not limited to, the warranties of fitness for particular purpose or merchantability, nor are any such representations implied with respect to the material set forth herein, and the publisher takes no responsibility with respect to such material. The publisher shall not be liable for any special, consequential, or exemplary damages resulting, in whole or part, from the readers' use of, or reliance upon, this material.

# Contents

▼   ▼   ▼   ▼   ▼   ▼   ▼

Preface . . . . . . . . . . . . . . . . . . . . . . . . . . . . . . . . . . . . . . . . . . . . . . xi

**Chapter 1** Introduction to Infection Control . . . . . . . . . . 1

Learning Objectives / 1
Key Terms / 1
Introduction / 1
History of Modern Infection Control / 2
Infection Control Becomes an Issue / 3
Current Perspective / 4
Statistics / 4
Infected Health Care Workers / 5
Conclusion / 7
Case Study 1.1 / 7
Questions for Discussion / 8
Worth Thinking About / 8
Bibliography / 8

**Chapter 2** Legal Issues . . . . . . . . . . . . . . . . . . . . . . . . . . . . . . . . . 9

Learning Objectives / 9
Key Terms / 9
Introduction / 10
Occupational Safety and Health Administration / 10
Ryan White CARE Act / 12
Americans with Disabilities Act / 14
Needlestick Prevention and Safety Act / 14
Agencies and Regulations / 15

Civil Liability / 16
Personal and Community Health / 17
Conclusion / 18
Case Study 2.1 / 19
Questions for Discussion / 20
Worth Thinking About / 20
Bibliography / 20

**Chapter 3** The Disease Process ..................... 22

Learning Objectives / 22
Key Terms / 22
Introduction / 23
Differentiation of Infectious and
   Communicable Diseases / 23
Direct and Indirect Exposure / 23
Causes of Disease / 23
Transmission / 26
Seroconversion / 27
Conclusion / 30
Case Study 3.1 / 30
Questions for Discussion / 31
Worth Thinking About / 32
Bibliography / 32

**Chapter 4** The Immune System ..................... 33

Learning Objectives / 33
Key Terms / 33
Introduction / 34
Structure of the Immune System / 35
Function of the Immune System / 37
The Immune Response / 38
Nonspecific Immunity / 39
Inflammatory Response / 40
      Phagocytosis / 41
      Other Types of Nonspecific Immunity / 42
Specific Immunity / 42
      Active and Passive Immunity / 43
Components of Specific Immunity / 43
      Antigens and Antibodies / 43
      B Lymphocytes / 44
      Humoral Immunity / 45

T Lymphocytes / 45
Cell-mediated Immunity / 45
Conclusion / 46
Case Study 4.1 / 46
Questions for Discussion / 47
Worth Thinking About / 47
Bibliography / 47

## Chapter 5 Diseases of Concern ...................... 48

Learning Objectives / 48
Key Terms / 49
Introduction / 51
Acquired Immunodeficiency Syndrome (AIDS) / 52
Amebiasis / 54
Anthrax (Woolsorters' Disease) / 55
Botulism / 56
Chlamydia / 57
Chickenpox / 58
Cryptosporidiosis / 60
Cytomegalovirus (CMV) / 62
*Escherichia coli (E. coli)* / 64
Gonorrhea / 65
Hantavirus Pulmonary Syndrome / 66
Hepatitis A / 68
Hepatitis B / 69
Hepatitis C / 70
Hepatitis Non-ABC / 72
Herpes Simplex 1 / 73
Herpes Simplex Type 2 (Genital Herpes) / 74
Influenza / 75
Legionellosis / 76
Lice (Pediculosis and Phthiriasis) / 77
Listeriosis / 79
Lyme Disease / 81
Measles (Rubeola, Hard Measles) / 82
Meningococcal Meningitis / 84
Mononucleosis / 85
Mumps / 86
Pertussis (Whooping Cough) / 87
Pneumonia / 89
Rabies / 91
Rocky Mountain Spotted Fever / 93
Rubella (German Measles) / 94

Salmonellosis / 97
Scabies / 98
Shigellosis / 100
Syphilis / 101
Tetanus / 103
Tuberculosis / 105
Case Study 5.1 / 107
Case Study 5.2 / 107
Questions for Discussion / 108
Worth Thinking About / 108
Bibliography / 109

**Chapter 6** Protection from Communicable Disease .. 111

Learning Objectives / 111
Key Terms / 112
Introduction / 112
Engineering Controls / 112
    Hand Washing Facilities / 113
    Biohazard Containers / 113
    Medical Devices / 114
    Other Concerns / 116
Safe Work Practices / 116
    Hand Washing / 117
    Handling and Using Sharps / 118
In-Hospital Isolation / 120
    Standard and Transmission-Based Precautions / 120
        Airborne Precautions / 121
        Droplet Precautions / 122
        Contact Precautions / 122
Out-of-Hospital Isolation / 123
Personal Protective Equipment / 123
    Gloves / 123
    Masks and Respirators / 124
    Eye Protection / 124
    Gowns and Protective Apparel / 126
    Uniforms / 126
Clean Up / 127
Personal Health / 128
    Physical Exams / 128
    Vaccinations / 128
    Hepatitis B Vaccine / 129
    Return to Work Authorization / 131
Conclusion / 131

Case Study 6.1 / 132
Questions for Discussion / 132
Worth Thinking About / 133
Bibliography / 133

# $\mathscr{C}$hapter 7 Exposure Determination .................. 134

Learning Objectives / 134
Key Terms / 134
Introduction / 134
Chain of Infection / 135
    Causative Agent / 135
    Source or Reservoir / 136
    Portal of Exit / 136
    Mode of Transmission / 136
    Portal of Entry / 136
    Susceptible Host / 136
Exposure in a Nutshell / 137
Airborne Exposure / 138
Conclusion / 139
Case Study 7.1 / 139
Questions for Discussion / 140
Worth Thinking About / 140
Bibliography / 140

# $\mathscr{C}$hapter 8 Post Exposure ........................... 141

Learning Objectives / 141
Key Terms / 141
Introduction / 142
First Aid / 142
Reporting / 142
Testing / 145
OSHA Reporting Requirements / 145
Return to Work / 146
Managing Stress / 146
    Counseling / 148
    Education / 148
    Physical Strategies / 148
Conclusion / 149
Case Study 8.1 / 149
Questions for Discussion / 150
Worth Thinking About / 150
Bibliography / 150

$\mathcal{A}$ppendix A Answers to
Questions for Discussion ................................151

Chapter 1 / 151
Chapter 2 / 151
Chapter 3 / 152
Chapter 4 / 153
Chapter 5 / 154
Chapter 6 / 155
Chapter 7 / 156
Chapter 8 / 157

$\mathcal{A}$ppendix B Discussion of Case Studies ........... 158

Case Study 1.1 / 158
Case Study 2.1 / 159
Case Study 3.1 / 159
Case Study 4.1 / 160
Case Study 5.1 / 161
Case Study 5.2 / 162
Case Study 6.1 / 163
Case Study 7.1 / 164
Case Study 8.1 / 165

$\mathcal{A}$ppendix C Glossary ............................166

Index ................................................. 175

# Preface

▼  ▼  ▼  ▼  ▼  ▼  ▼

## INTRODUCTION

*Basic Infection Control for Health Care Providers* is designed to provide current, relevant information about infection control and infectious disease. Health care providers from any discipline and at any experience level will benefit from the practical advice contained in this book. Whether you are just starting out as a student in one of the many health related professions or are an experienced health care provider, this book will give you the information you need to protect yourself from infectious disease and protect yourself from legal repercussions.

This book may also prove useful for others who have occupational exposure to blood and other potentially infectious material. Day care workers, police officers, firefighters, factory workers, and tattoo artists may all benefit from the material contained herein. Regardless of your occupation, this book will serve as a practical reference and a helpful tool.

Infection control is a dynamic field. Practically every month discoveries are made, court decisions are formed, and outbreaks are tracked. The future of infection control is exciting. A vaccine is currently being developed for hepatitis C, a disease we have been aware of for only a few years. In recent years, we have seen infectious agents used as weapons of mass destruction against civilians. Though these attacks have not been perpetrated against United States citizens on U.S. soil, the federal government has taken seriously the threat of terrorist activity and has developed plans for defense from such an attack. Health care providers must be aware of these agents. Even as you read this, the Centers for Disease Control and Prevention are monitoring emerging infectious diseases in an attempt to prevent outbreaks. Changes in this field come often, and have far-reaching consequences.

## DEVELOPMENT OF THIS BOOK

Several years ago I was given the opportunity to teach an infection control class for a multi-disciplined group of health care providers. The challenge, I soon discovered, was finding an appropriate book for the class. Infection control books were available, but none that provided the breadth and depth of information that I wished to cover.

The solution, though not an optimal one, was to photocopy my many pages of notes for the students, adding to the material as I discovered topics that needed to be covered. This packet of notes developed into a small, self-published booklet which, after many classes of student review, served as a foundation for *Basic Infection Control for Health Care Providers*. Much of the material in this book is a result of student critique of my self-published book.

This material has been class tested over a period of five years and has been fine-tuned to fit the needs of anyone from entry-level students to seasoned professionals in any of the many health care disciplines. The content of this book was developed with the curricula of several health care professions in mind, including the new Department of Transportation EMT Intermediate and

Paramedic curriculum. Input from faculty of nursing and paramedic programs was also very helpful in the development of this book. Other disciplines, including those in the following list, were represented in the development of this book:

- chiropractors
- day care providers
- dentists, dental assistants, and hygienists
- emergency medical services personnel
- fire service personnel
- industrial safety personnel
- laboratory personnel
- nursing home workers
- nursing personnel
- occupational therapists
- physical therapy personnel
- physicians
- radiological technologists
- respiratory therapists and technicians
- shelter workers
- sports medicine personnel, coaches, and trainers
- teachers and school personnel
- workers in business and industry

## ORGANIZATION OF THE TEXT

*Basic Infection Control for Health Care Providers* includes eight chapters and three appendixes intended to provide the reader with a well-rounded package of materials in a convenient format.

Each chapter opens with a list of learning objectives. Information about these objectives is found in the text in a clear, concise manner. Terminology that may be unfamiliar to the student is highlighted within the text as bold type and is included in the glossary. Questions for discussion are found at the end of each chapter, giving the reader the opportunity for self-evaluation. Additional questions that may be worth thinking about are listed for enrichment. Key points within the chapter are reinforced with a case study intended to stimulate discussion and critical thinking. Reflect and Consider questions give the reader the opportunity to analyze the case and its implications. Alert boxes throughout each chapter alert the reader to situations about which health care providers should be aware.

Chapter 5 may be used as lecture material or as a reference for health care providers. Extensive information on over 35 diseases of concern to the health care provider is included.

Appendix A offers answers for each of the Questions for Discussion and Appendix B includes discussion of each of the case studies. A glossary that defines more than 200 terms is included as the final appendix.

## FEATURES OF THE BOOK

This book offers the following features:

*Learning Objectives*—Each chapter opens with a list of learning objectives that are the substance of the chapter content.

*Key Terms*—A listing of key terms alerts the reader to terms that may be new or unfamiliar. These terms are bolded in the text and defined in the glossary.

*Case Studies*—Case studies are used to illustrate key points and promote critical thinking.

*Questions for Discussion*—Questions are based on learning objectives and answers may be found within the chapter or in Appendix A.

*Alerts*—Alerts are used to call attention to something about which the health care provider should be aware.

These features, coupled with the content applicable to any of the health care disciplines, make this book one that is as comprehensive as it is easy to read.

# SUPPLEMENT PACKAGE

The *Instructor Manual* is designed to complement *Basic Infection Control for Health Care Providers* and create an integrated teaching package that will provide the instructor with resources needed to conduct an infection control course that exceeds OSHA standards.

The *Instructor Manual* includes:
- Annotated outline with suggested exercises
- Sample course agendas
- Course outline
- Materials for exercises and role-plays
- Flash cards

# ABOUT THE AUTHOR

Mike Kennamer is a graduate of the paramedic program at Gadsden State Community College in Gadsden, Alabama. He holds a B.S. in public safety administration from Athens State University in Athens, Alabama, and an M.P.A. from Jacksonville State University in Jacksonville, Alabama.

Mr. Kennamer serves as director of emergency medical services at Northeast Alabama Community College in Rainsville, Alabama and is a charter member of the National Association of EMS Educators. He serves on the Alabama EMS Education Committee and has been active on several Alabama College System committees.

# $\mathcal{A}$CKNOWLEDGMENTS

I wish to thank the following reviewers who provided valuable input on the content and structure of this book:
Ann Sims, RN, BSN
Albuquerque Technical-Vocational Institute
Albuquerque, NM

Rich Bronson, M.Ed., EMT-P
Oklahoma State Department of Health
Grove, OK

Nancy Bourgeois, RN, BSN
Office of Public Health
Baton Rouge, LA

I also wish to thank the many students and colleagues who have reviewed one or more chapters, made suggestions on content, or simply put up with my incessant questions about what should, and should not, be included in a book on infection control for health care providers.

The Delmar team was wonderful to work with. *Basic Infection Control for Health Care Providers* was initally signed by acquisitions editor Doris Smith. Doris was a tremendous help and incredibly patient in answering question after question as I wrote the manuscript. Later, Maureen Muncaster aptly took control of the project and saw it through to completion. Thanks, Maureen, for "adopting" my project.

Production editor, Jim Zayicek, was great to work with and provided all the answers to many questions. Though I didn't have frequent contact with executive editor, Cathy Esperti, or executive marketing manager, Dawn Gerrain, it was apparent that their work and the work of the other Delmar folks behind the scenes made this project possible.

Jill Korznat, editorial assistant, was a tremendous help as she cheerfully fielded my frequent emails and constant questions. Thanks, Jill, for keeping me on track. Special thanks is also due to Judi Orozco at TDB Publishing Services for transforming the manuscript into the book you are now holding.

Finally, I would be deeply amiss if I did not recognize the importance of the support of my family while writing this book. My wife, Trisha, was a tremendous help during the entire process. Whether she was working on the glossary, writing case studies, or just bouncing ideas around, her input and partnership in the process was invaluable. My three sons, Devin, Cody, and Lane, were very patient (and sometimes even quiet) when Dad was working. Devin was very helpful in the development of the games and activities for the *Instructor Manual* and in organizing the art manuscript. Cody and Lane always helped me keep things in perspective and offered a hug and a smile when needed.

## FEEDBACK

The author is interested in hearing from anyone who would like to offer suggestions or constructive criticism for future editions of this book. Please feel free to contact the author through Delmar or directly by email at kennamerm@nacc.cc.al.us.

# Chapter 1
# Introduction to Infection Control

▼  ▼  ▼  ▼  ▼  ▼  ▼

## LEARNING OBJECTIVES

After completing this chapter, the reader should be able to:

- discuss the history of infection control.
- recognize and discuss modern infection control threats.
- list three key figures in the development of modern infection control.
- recognize and discuss infection control as a rapidly changing field.

## KEY TERMS

- acquired immunodeficiency syndrome
- hepatitis B (HBV)
- hepatitis C (HCV)
- occupational exposure
- tuberculosis (TB)
- virulence

## INTRODUCTION

Infection control is a rapidly changing field. This book is an overview of how the health care provider who is at risk of **occupational exposure** to blood and/or body fluid may be protected from contracting a communicable disease. Persons reading this book should realize that because changes occur rapidly, the instructor of this course is an important resource for the most up-to-date information.

## HISTORY OF MODERN INFECTION CONTROL

Modern infection control ideas originated in Vienna, Austria in the mid-1800s when a physician, Ignaz Semmelweis, discovered that hand washing seemed to decrease the incidence of death due to infection following childbirth. By observing simple hand washing procedures, the death rate related to infection decreased from 18% to 1% in Semmelweis' hospital. Although Semmelweis was excited with his discovery, the concept of washing hands before and after medical procedures was not routinely practiced until much later.

Unfortunately, Semmelweis' colleagues were not as enthusiastic about his discovery. His hospital censured him and reduced his privileges. When he reported his findings to the Medical Society of Vienna, he met enough resistance to lead him to his native Budapest. There he was committed to an insane asylum, and died of an infection similar to those he had tried to prevent in Austria.

During about the same period, French scientist Louis Pasteur created his germ theory. A background in physics and chemistry led Pasteur to approach the study of microbial life in a different way. Pasteur believed that microbes can bring about significant transformations in organic matter—transformations that are very selective and specific in their activities. Pasteur also discovered anaerobic life when practical application of his germ theory proved that, in the absence of air, sugar was converted to butyric acid. Not only did his different approach open new doors in the field of microbiology, it also led to the development of the process of pasteurization—a technique of controlled heating for the preservation of various food products.

Scottish surgeon Joseph Lister expanded Pasteur's germ theory by using cotton wool and bandages treated with carbolic acid to dress surgical wounds. It was Lister who discovered that infection could be prevented by covering wounds and using antiseptic agents. Like Semmelweis, the efficacy of his work was demonstrated by a post-surgery mortality rate that decreased from 50% to 15%. And like Semmelweis, he initially experienced great resistance from the medical community. Lister, however, persevered and became famous during his lifetime. He performed surgery on Queen Victoria and opened the way for techniques of modern surgery.

Just as Semmelweis had trouble convincing his colleagues to wash their hands, health care providers as recently as several years ago were not convinced of the necessity of observing standard precautions against communicable disease. What do you think it took to convince health care providers to observe precautions against communicable disease? See if you agree with the analysis in the following section.

## INFECTION CONTROL BECOMES AN ISSUE

In the 1980s, a disease called **acquired immunodeficiency syndrome (AIDS)** was introduced to the American public. Although early reports sparked little interest, people began to take note when celebrities and sports figures became infected with the disease. As the disease spread throughout the country, persons with occupational exposure to blood started to routinely wear gloves and other protective equipment. Organizations set standards and the United States government began work on legislation that would protect America's health care workers.

**ALERT**

Diseases other than hepatitis and human immunodeficiency virus (HIV) pose a risk for health care providers. Always protect yourself from all infectious and communicable disease.

## CURRENT PERSPECTIVE

Today communicable disease is taken seriously. Employees take the initiative to better protect themselves and employers meet stringent standards imposed by the federal government to ensure a safe workplace.

AIDS remains a formidable disease. There is no vaccine and no cure. Other diseases like **tuberculosis (TB)**, **hepatitis B (HBV)**, and **hepatitis C (HCV)** continue to affect health care providers and remain considerable health risks. Currently, five times as many Americans are infected with HCV than are infected with HIV. Due to the **virulence** of hepatitis and its ability to survive outside the confines of the human body, health care providers are at risk of occupational exposure.

## STATISTICS

The Centers for Disease Control and Prevention (CDC) estimate that 33.6 million people worldwide are infected with HIV, the virus that causes AIDS. Between 650,000 and 900,000 of these are U.S. residents and, according to CDC estimates, up to 200,000 of these may be unaware that they are infected.

Hepatitis B emerged as a significant health risk in the 1980s. Though public education and an effective vaccine have contributed to decreasing numbers of persons infected with hepatitis B virus (HBV), the CDC estimates that 128,000 U.S. residents become infected each year. Hepatitis B is very environmentally resistant and can survive for long periods of time, even outside the body.

Currently hepatitis C is the most common chronic bloodborne infection in the U.S. An estimated 3.9 million Americans have been infected with HCV. Worldwide, it is estimated that 170 million have been infected. According to the CDC, most of these persons may not be aware of their infection because they are not clinically ill. Researchers are working on a vaccine for HCV, which is expected to be available by 2004.

Other diseases may pose a risk to the health care provider. Tuberculosis (TB), which was once the leading cause of death in the United States, was thought to be a disease of the past until 1984 when it began to make a comeback. Many attribute the comeback of tuberculosis to public apathy and failure to vaccinate.

## INFECTED HEALTH CARE WORKERS

As of December 31, 1999, approximately 5.1% (22,218) of the adults in the U.S. reported to have AIDS had been employed in a health care field. The job type is known for 94% of these workers as listed in Figure 1-1. Overall, 74% of these health care workers with AIDS have died. Of these 22,218 infected health care workers, the Centers for Disease Control and Prevention (CDC) is aware of only 56 who have been documented as having been infected with HIV following a known occupational exposure. The overwhelming majority of these workers were exposed through cuts or needlesticks. Twenty-five have developed AIDS. Figure 1-2 lists the job titles of those with infection secondary to documented occupational exposure.

| | |
|---|---|
| Nurses | 4,856 |
| Health aides | 4,859 |
| Technicians | 2,933 |
| Physicians | 1,691 |
| Therapists | 1,010 |
| Dental workers | 467 |
| Paramedics | 424 |
| Surgeons | 114 |

FIGURE 1-1 Health care workers infected with HIV. (Source: Centers for Disease Control and Prevention.)

| | |
|---|---|
| Nurses | 23 |
| Lab workers | 19 |
| Physicians | 6 |
| Surgical technicians | 2 |
| Dialysis technicians | 1 |
| Respiratory therapists | 1 |
| Health aides | 1 |
| Embalmers/morgue technicians | 1 |
| Housekeepers/maintenance | 2 |

FIGURE 1-2 Job titles of health care providers with infection secondary to documented occupational exposure. (Source: Centers for Disease Control and Prevention.)

The CDC is also aware of 136 cases of HIV infection among health care workers where infection after specific exposure was not documented but no specific risk factors other than occupational exposure were known.

Current studies show that the average risk of HIV infection after a needlestick or cut exposure to HIV-infected blood is 0.3% (about one in 300) where risk after exposure of the mouth, eye, nose, or skin to HIV-infected blood is 0.1% (about one in 1,000) or less.

Since the hepatitis B vaccine has become available, the number of occupational infections has decreased sharply. In the period from 1985 to 1996 there was a decrease of approximately 90%. The risk, however, remains as approximately 800 health care workers become infected with HBV each year due to occupational exposure.

Though the CDC has not yet estimated the number of health care workers occupationally infected with hepatitis C, studies reveal that 1% of hospital health care workers have evidence of HCV infection. This figure is somewhat less than the estimated 1.8% of the U.S. general population that is infected with HCV.

## CONCLUSION

All health care providers have an obligation to learn about infectious disease in an effort to protect themselves and their patients. The remainder of this book will serve as a basis for that knowledge.

## CASE STUDY 1.1

Your patient is a 15-year-old female who became ill while attending a cheerleading camp. She now complains of nausea, vomiting, abdominal cramps, and bloody diarrhea. You learn that this and other campers frequently filled water bottles with ice from an open barrel located in the dormitory lobby. This barrel was lined with a garbage bag and campers report that they frequently dipped their water bottles, hands, arms, and heads into the ice. According to her fellow campers, debris was frequently seen floating in the ice barrels.

*(continued)*

REFLECT AND CONSIDER

➤ What is the likely source of your patient's illness?
➤ How could this exposure have been prevented?
➤ How could education have prevented this exposure?

## QUESTIONS FOR DISCUSSION

1. What one disease has increased awareness of infection control the most in recent years?
2. What simple infection control procedure helped Dr. Ignaz Semmelweis save a number of lives in the 1800s?
3. List three pioneers in the field of infection control.
4. List at least three diseases that should concern health care workers today.

## WORTH THINKING ABOUT

• Try to recall the first time you heard about AIDS. Have you experienced prejudices against those with AIDS or other communicable diseases? Why?
• Have you ever cared for a person with AIDS? Did you take more precautions with this patient than you normally do? Why?

## BIBLIOGRAPHY

Coughlin, C., & Craft, A. (2000, March). Hepatitis C: The silent epidemic. *Journal of Emergency Medical Services* 25(3): 114–129.

Dubos, R. J., & Hirsch, J. G. (1965). *Bacterial and mycotic infections of man.* Philadelphia, PA: J. B. Lippincott.

Shimeld, L. A., & Rodgers, A. T. (1999). *Essentials of diagnostic microbiology.* Albany, NY: Delmar.

# $\mathscr{C}$hapter 2
# Legal Issues

▼   ▼   ▼   ▼   ▼   ▼   ▼

## $\mathscr{L}$EARNING OBJECTIVES

After completing this chapter, the reader should be able to:

- list at least four things required by the OSHA bloodborne pathogen standard.
- explain the importance of meeting national standards.
- discuss the intent of the Ryan White CARE Act.
- describe the role of the designated officer.
- list at least three organizations that are considered leaders in infection control issues.
- describe reasons for learning more about infection control.
- list the components of a successful negligence lawsuit.

## $\mathscr{K}$EY TERMS

- Americans with Disabilities Act (ADA)
- breach of duty
- category I employee
- Centers for Disease Control and Prevention (CDC)
- civil liability
- damages
- designated officer

- duty to act
- exposure control plan
- National Fire Academy (NFA)
- National Fire Protection Association (NFPA)
- negligence
- notification by request
- Occupational Safety and Health Administration (OSHA)
- proximate cause
- routine notification
- Ryan White CARE Act of 1990
- standard of care

## INTRODUCTION

This chapter briefs the reader on three major reasons people learn about infection control. First, administrative law requires that employees at risk of exposure to blood and body fluid receive training on infection control issues. Second, the employee who fails to meet national standards may be subject to civil action. And third, the employee should want to learn about protection from exposure to communicable disease. This education will not only protect employees, but will also protect families and the community at large.

## OCCUPATIONAL SAFETY AND HEALTH ADMINISTRATION

In 1991, the Occupational Safety and Health Administration (OSHA), under authority of Congress, set the rule for occupational exposure to bloodborne pathogens in title 29, part 1910 of the Code of Federal Regulations. This rule was a landmark in the development of infection control programs in the United

States and set the wheels in motion for the development of infection control training as it is known today.

This rule identified health care providers and emergency response personnel as **category I employees** who are at the greatest risk of occupational exposure to communicable disease. It also mandated each employer with category I employees to develop an **exposure control plan** and to offer hepatitis B vaccinations at no charge to the employee. Standards on personal protective equipment (PPE), recordkeeping, training, and work practices were also developed and carry the weight of law. Required exposure control plan contents are listed in Figure 2-1.

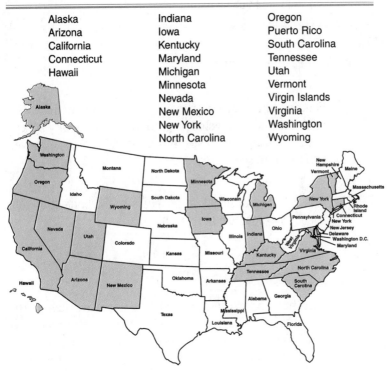

| | | |
|---|---|---|
| Alaska | Indiana | Oregon |
| Arizona | Iowa | Puerto Rico |
| California | Kentucky | South Carolina |
| Connecticut | Maryland | Tennessee |
| Hawaii | Michigan | Utah |
| | Minnesota | Vermont |
| | Nevada | Virgin Islands |
| | New Mexico | Virginia |
| | New York | Washington |
| | North Carolina | Wyoming |

FIGURE 2-1 States and territories with OSHA-approved plans. (Source: Occupational Safety and Health Administration.)

Each agency's exposure control plan should be tailored for the agency. Common components of the plan should include:
- Purpose
- Scope (To whom does the plan apply?)
- Exposure determination
- Post exposure protocols
- Standard operating procedures
- Roles and responsibilities
- Personal protective equipment
- Training standards
- Health maintenance
- Engineering controls
- Compliance and quality monitoring

**FIGURE 2-2** Exposure control plan contents. (Source: Occupational Safety and Health Administration.)

Federal law requires that states comply with OSHA regulations or develop a plan that meets or exceeds OSHA standards. To see if your state has an approved OSHA plan, see Figure 2-2.

**ALERT**

It is your responsibility to be aware of the content of your agency's exposure control plan.

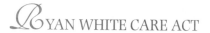 RYAN WHITE CARE ACT

Another important law for health care workers is the **Ryan White Comprehensive AIDS Resources Emergency (CARE) Act of 1990**. This law, reauthorized in 1996, gives employees the right to learn if they were exposed to infectious disease while caring for a patient. To learn more about Ryan White, see Figure 2-3.

*"I always knew it would take a long time to educate people, but I never knew it would take this long."*

*Ryan White*

The day after Christmas in 1984, thirteen-year-old Ryan White was told by his mother that he had AIDS. A hemophiliac, White became infected through a transfusion of HIV-tainted blood and later became an important force in educating the public about AIDS.

A young boy with a misunderstood disease, Ryan White was often the victim of fear and ignorance. Children in school called him names and ostracized him. Adults refused to shake hands with his family at church and someone even fired a bullet into his house. Frightened parents asked that Ryan be kept out of school and Ryan sued to secure his right to public education. Though he won the suit, he still felt uncomfortable in his home town of Kokomo, Indiana so he moved to Cicero, Indiana where he was welcomed at Hamilton Heights High School.

It was during this legal battle that Ryan White decided to dedicate the remainder of his life to educating the public about AIDS. Until his death just a few years later, Ryan White captivated America with his knowledge of and courage in dealing with his disease.

Ryan White's contribution to public education about AIDS was essential in building a foundation of understanding and helping to dispel many myths about the disease. This contribution prompted Congress to name the most comprehensive AIDS legislation to date after Ryan White.

FIGURE 2-3  Ryan White.

The law requires each employer to name a **designated officer** to serve as a liaison between the employee and the physician after an exposure. Notification takes place in one of two ways.

**Routine notification** is provided by the treating facility or hospital to employees exposed to a patient who is found to be infected with an airborne communicable disease. Emergency response personnel who transport a patient who is later discovered to have an airborne communicable disease are automatically considered to have been exposed. Since the ambulance is an enclosed space, it is assumed that anyone within that space is likely to have been exposed. Other health care providers who care for a patient in an enclosed space should receive routine notification as well.

**Notification by request** is made by any employee who is potentially exposed to a communicable disease while providing patient care. This request is made by the employee and coordinated through the designated officer.

## AMERICANS WITH DISABILITIES ACT

The **Americans with Disabilities Act (ADA)** is intended to prohibit discrimination against persons with disabilities. The act specifically notes "contagious disease" as a qualifying disability which ensures that employees who contract a communicable disease will not be discriminated against.

## NEEDLESTICK PREVENTION AND SAFETY ACT

The Centers for Disease Control and Prevention (CDC) estimate that more than 380,000 percutaneous injuries from contaminated sharps occur each year among United States health care workers in the hospital setting. With this many or more percutaneous injuries from contaminated sharps occurring outside the hospitals, Congress sponsored the Needlestick Prevention and Safety Act of 2000. This act, which enjoyed strong bipartisan support, was signed into law on November 6, 2000. Its purpose is to protect health care providers from accidental needlesticks by requiring employers to solicit input from non-managerial employees, responsible for direct patient care, in the identification, evaluation, and selection of effective engineering and work practice controls. Specific provisions of this act include an emphasis on selection, training, and use of safer medical devices and the development of a sharps injury log for better surveillance of percutaneous injuries from contaminated sharps.

This log is required in addition to the OSHA 200 log (300 log beginning January 1, 2002) and must contain the following items:

- the type and brand of device involved in the incident
- the work area or department where the incident occurred
- an explanation of how the incident occurred

Companies who have employed no more than ten employees at any time during the preceding calendar year are not required to maintain this log. The information on this log must be kept for five years and maintained in such a way as to protect the confidentiality of the injured employee.

## AGENCIES AND REGULATIONS

Several agencies have established standards for infection control. The **Centers for Disease Control and Prevention (CDC)** has been instrumental in publishing standards for infection control and in establishing guidelines for standard precautions. The CDC tracks selected diseases and monitors for trends in the appearance of diseases in a particular area. Through research, education, and extensive publishing in the area of infectious disease, the CDC has emerged as an incredible resource for those who wish to learn more about infection control.

The National Fire Academy (NFA) has promoted the educational aspect of infection control and was among the first to publish texts on the 1991 bloodborne pathogen standard. The National Fire Protection Association (NFPA) was one of the first national agencies to publish standards on infection control. Although written for fire departments, many of these standards are applicable to other employers and have been used as a guide in the development of standards in other fields.

## &#x1D49E;IVIL LIABILITY

Standards set forth by national organizations may not carry the weight of law, but one should take these standards as seriously as if they were federal law.

Employers and/or employees may be found guilty of civil liability if damages occur as a result of not meeting national standards. Although no law is broken, they may be found negligent if they do not meet standards that would be met by another reasonable person in a similar position.

There are four components needed to prove that a health care provider was negligent. These four components of negligence are explained as follows:

- **Duty to act**—Before a person may be considered negligent, he/she must have a legal duty to provide care. This duty to act obligates the caregiver to treat the patient with the same standard of care that would be offered by another reasonable caregiver of the same level of training.

- **Breach of duty**—A breach of duty means that the caregiver did not meet his/her obligation in some way. This may be inappropriate care, abandonment, or care that is either above or below the caregiver's expected level of care.

- **Damages**—When a patient has experienced monetary loss, injury, or death, she or her family is said to have experienced damages. Damages may be tangible, like loss of income, or intangible, like loss of vision.

- **Proximate cause**—The final component, which must be proven to show negligence, is proximate cause. That is, that the damages resulted from the caregiver's breach of duty. Even if there are damages and a breach of duty, negligence is not proven until it can be shown that the damages were caused by the breach of duty.

Though we usually think of breach of duty as inappropriate action or treatment, it is possible that failure to meet national standards may constitute negligence when damages occur as a result of that failure. Case Study 2.1 illustrates this point.

## PERSONAL AND COMMUNITY HEALTH

Health care providers should, even if not required by law, seek to stay current with infection control training as a method of promoting personal health and the health of their families. Knowledge of infection control procedures and protection measures may contribute to a longer and more productive career and life.

Employees also have a responsibility to the community to learn how to minimize the possibility for cross contamination from patient-to-patient and from employee-to-patient. Health care providers who have young children should take an active role in educating neighborhood children of the importance of hand washing and the dangers of behavior that may lead to disease spread.

# Conclusion

There are a number of good reasons for participating in infection control training. Some people see legal repercussions as a good reason, while others are motivated by the desire to protect themselves and their families. Whatever your reason for taking this training, it is important that you stay up-to-date on infection control issues.

OSHA requires training each year to keep health care providers up-to-date. Don't depend on taking one course or reading one book to keep you updated for life. Infection control is a dynamic field and should be revisited often, as scientific discoveries are made and legal cases are upheld or overturned. This is an area where lifelong learning could prove to be a lifesaving experience.

## CASE STUDY 2.1

Your local hospital adopts a new technique for cardiopulmonary resuscitation (CPR), which it uses to replace the standards set forth by national organizations. Because your hospital administrator believes it best to perform a pulse check before opening the airway, the traditional order of ABC (Airway-Breathing-Circulation) is changed to CAB (Circulation-Airway-Breathing). This change from the national standards may never cause a problem until a law suit is filed.

If a suit is filed in this case, the attorney for the plaintiff may attempt to show that:

- hospital personnel had a duty to act.
- there was a breach of duty in that hospital personnel strayed from national standards.
- damages occurred.
- damages were caused as a result of that deviation from national standards.

The attorney may argue, in this case, that brain damage occurred because there was a delay in opening the airway and ventilating the patient.

Though this case is totally fictitious and unrealistic, it should help you realize why adherence to national standards is so important.

### REFLECT AND CONSIDER

> Regardless of whether the hospital wins the suit, it may spend significant sums of money to defend the actions of the administrator. How can hospital administration prevent such lawsuits from occurring in the future?

## QUESTIONS FOR DISCUSSION

1. List three things required by OSHA regarding infection control.
2. If your state is not an OSHA state, why should you conform to OSHA regulations?
3. What is the intent of the Ryan White CARE Act?
4. Explain routine notification.
5. Explain notification by request.
6. What is the role of the designated officer in an organization?

## WORTH THINKING ABOUT

- Consider the responsibility you feel in taking this course.

## BIBLIOGRAPHY

AIDS Action Council. (1996, May 20). "*Clinton signs Ryan White CARE Act Reauthorization Bill.*" (media release). http://www.thebody.com/aac/may2096.html.

AIDS 101.com Internet site: http://www.aids101.com.

Centers for Disease Control. (1989, June 23). Guidelines for prevention of transmission of human immunodeficiency virus and hepatitis B virus to healthcare and public safety workers. *Morbidity and Mortality Weekly Report 38, no. S-6.*

Channaiah, D. *The Ryan White story: A shift from confusion, fear, and ignorance to acceptance and new-found knowledge of AIDS.* http://www.engl.virginia.edu/~enwr1016/dc5k/aids.html.

National Fire Academy. (1992). *Infection control for emergency response personnel: The supervisor's role.* Emmitsburg, MD: Author.

Nielson, R. P. (2000). *OSHA regulations and guidelines: A guide for health care providers.* Albany, NY: Delmar.

U.S. Department of Labor, Occupational Safety and Health Administration. (1991, Dec. 6). *Occupational exposure to bloodborne pathogens.* CFR 1910.1030, Final Rule.

U.S. Department of Labor, Occupational Safety and Health Administration. (1992). *Occupational exposure to bloodborne pathogens: Precautions for emergency responders.* OSHA 3130.

U.S. Department of Labor, Occupational Safety and Health Administration. (1999, Nov. 5). *Enforcement procedures for the occupational exposure to bloodborne pathogens.* Directive no. CPL 2-2.44D.

United States Fire Administration. (1992). *Guide to developing and managing an emergency service infection control program.* Washington, DC: Author.

Wilcox, W., (Ed.). (1998). *Public health sourcebook, Health Reference Series,* (54). Omnigraphics, Inc.

# Chapter 3
## The Disease Process

▼  ▼  ▼  ▼  ▼  ▼  ▼

## LEARNING OBJECTIVES

After completing this chapter, the reader should be able to:

- differentiate between infectious and communicable disease.
- describe at least two ways disease is spread.
- list at least four causes of infectious disease.
- list the stages of an infectious disease.
- explain the principles of seroconversion.

## KEY TERMS

- airborne transmission
- bacteria
- bloodborne transmission
- casual contact
- communicable disease
- fungus
- helminths
- household contact
- incubation period
- infectious disease
- other potentially infectious material (OPIM)
- parasitic
- protozoans

- rickettsia
- saprophytic
- seroconversion
- sexual transmission
- sexually transmitted disease (STD)
- vector borne transmission
- virus
- window phase

## INTRODUCTION

The material presented in this chapter forms a brief overview of the disease process. By understanding how the disease process works, health care providers can better protect themselves from infectious disease.

## DIFFERENTIATION OF INFECTIOUS AND COMMUNICABLE DISEASES

In the study of the disease process, it is important to differentiate between infectious disease and communicable disease (Figure 3-1). An **infectious disease** is one that results from an invasion of a host from a disease-producing organism. This organism may be in the form of a virus, bacteria, fungus, or parasite. A **communicable disease** is an infectious disease that may be transmitted from one person to another. Employees at risk of occupational exposure to blood and body fluids should be especially concerned with human immunodeficiency virus (HIV), hepatitis B virus (HBV), hepatitis C virus (HCV), and tuberculosis (TB).

## DIRECT AND INDIRECT EXPOSURE

Exposure to communicable disease may occur by direct person-to-person contact through events such as sexual

| Infectious diseases that are communicable | Infectious diseases that are not communicable |
|---|---|
| • Hepatitis B | • Anthrax |
| • Influenza | • Botulism |
| • Chlamydia | • Salmonellosis |
| • Measles | • Lyme disease |

FIGURE 3-1  Infectious versus communicable disease.

contact or a contaminated needlestick. Exposure may also be indirect through handling soiled linens or touching a contaminated object.

## CAUSES OF DISEASE

While health care providers are often concerned with viral and bacterial diseases, one should realize that there are a number of other causes of infectious disease (Figure 3-2). Fungi, protozoa, and rickettsia are all known to cause infectious disease. Descriptions of each of the main causes of infectious disease follow.

**Bacteria** are living microorganisms that can produce disease in a host. Bacteria can self-reproduce and some may produce toxins that are harmful to their host. Bacteria are also capable of living outside the host. Diseases like bacterial meningitis, tetanus, food poisoning, tuberculosis, and syphilis are caused by bacteria.

**Viruses** are microorganisms that reside within other living cells and cannot reproduce outside a living cell. Viruses like HIV, HBV, and influenza may pose risks to those with occupational exposure.

| Cause | Examples |
|-------|----------|
| Virus | Influenza, HIV, HBV |
| Bacteria | Tetanus, syphilis, tuberculosis |
| Helminth | .Pinworms, tapeworms |
| Fungus | Tinea, dhobie itch |
| Protozoa | Malaria, dysentery |
| Rickettsia | Rocky Mountain Spotted Fever, typhus |

FIGURE 3-2 Causes of infectious disease.

A fungus is a plantlike organism that grows as single cells (e.g., yeast) or as multicellular colonies (e.g., mold). Since fungi do not contain chlorophyll, they depend on a parasitic or saprophytic existence. Examples of fungal infectious diseases include tinea (ringworm) and dhobie itch.

Protozoans are the simplest organisms in the animal kingdom. Many are single-celled, though some colonize. Examples of protozoal infections include malaria, dysentery, and sleeping sickness.

Rickettsias are parasitical creatures who depend on living cells for growth. Usually transmitted by fleas, ticks, lice, and mites, infectious diseases caused by rickettsiae include Rocky Mountain Spotted Fever and several forms of typhus.

Helminths (worms) may also cause infectious disease. While many worms are not parasitic, parasitic worms like pinworms and tapeworms may be acquired by eating under-cooked meat.

# TRANSMISSION

When a communicable disease is passed from one person to another, a series of events takes place, creating a chain of infection (Figure 3-3). The first of these events is transmission, which may be airborne, bloodborne, or vector borne.

**Airborne transmission** is typically accomplished through droplets in a sneeze or cough. These aerosolized droplets travel through the air and are inhaled through the respiratory system or absorbed through mucous membranes. Tuberculosis is a common airborne transmissible disease.

**ALERT**

It may be difficult to determine exposure to airborne transmissible disease. Health care providers should observe standard precautions when caring for any patient with a cough or sneeze.

**Bloodborne transmission** takes place when infected blood or blood-containing body fluid is introduced into the body of another person. Common ways this is accomplished are through needlesticks, splashing into the mucous membranes, or blood contacting nonintact skin.

**Vector borne transmission** is transmission of a disease-causing organism through an outside source, or a vector. This includes a mosquito that carries malaria or a tick that carries Rocky Mountain Spotted Fever.

**Sexual transmission** is transmission of a disease through sexual contact with an infected person. Transmission is usually accomplished through the contact of infected body fluids with mucous membranes. **Sexually transmitted diseases (STDs)** include gonorrhea, syphilis, and genital herpes.

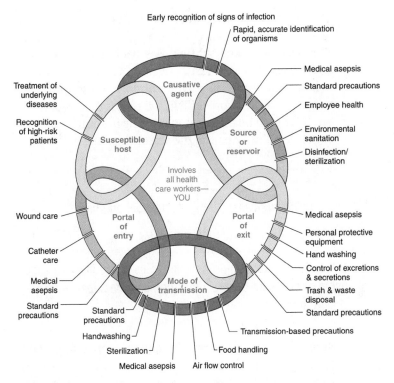

FIGURE 3-3 Chain of infection. As with any chain, if one link is broken, the infection can not be spread. This figure shows ways health care providers can break each link in the chain of infection.

Some diseases are transmitted person-to-person by **casual contact** or **household contact**. This includes close body-to-body contact, sleeping in the same bed, and sharing hairbrushes or combs. Children who become infested with lice or scabies frequently catch them through casual contact at school.

## SEROCONVERSION

Once a disease is introduced into the body, a period of time elapses before a blood test will read "positive."

This process of converting from a "negative" to a "positive" blood test is called seroconversion (Figure 3-4). The period of time that elapses between an exposure and a positive blood test is referred to as the window phase. The duration of the window phase may vary considerably from one individual to another, depending on the overall health, response of the immune system in the infected person, and the strength of the pathogen.

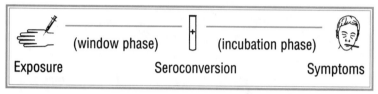

(window phase)      (incubation phase)

Exposure                   Seroconversion              Symptoms

FIGURE 3-4 Seroconversion progression. This figure illustrates the relationship of exposure to seroconversion and the appearance of the first symptoms.

Symptoms do not normally appear immediately with seroconversion. The time that passes between seroconversion and the appearance of symptoms is called the incubation period. For hepatitis B (HBV) this period may be up to two hundred days. The incubation period for human immunodeficiency virus (HIV) may be as long as ten years. Refer to Figure 3-5 for a summary of the possible stages of infectious disease.

It is important that both the patient and the caregiver realize that a single negative blood test and lack of immediate symptoms do not necessarily mean that a person is free from a disease. Follow-up testing at prescribed intervals is highly recommended.

The importance of protecting oneself from exposure to blood and other potentially infectious material (OPIM) is apparent when we realize that the carrier of HIV may display no signs or symptoms for up to ten years.

| Latent period | Period after infection when an infectious agent can not be transmitted to another host |
|---|---|
| Communicable period | Period after infection when an infectious agent can be transmitted to another host |
| Incubation period | Time between exposure and onset of symptoms |
| Window phase | Period where antigen is present but seroconversion has not yet taken place |
| Disease period | Time between onset of symptoms and resolution of symptoms |

FIGURE 3-5 Stages of infectious disease.

Consider this example of why knowledge of seroconversion is important to health care providers.

Nancy, a registered nurse, is attending her son's Little League baseball game when another child is struck in the face by a batted ball, resulting in profuse bleeding from the nose and mouth. The patient appears in good health, but Nancy has no gloves readily available. She helps control the bleeding without the benefit of personal protective equipment (PPE). Though the child's young age and apparent state of health may make Nancy feel comfortable treating him without personal protective equipment, she may be placing herself in danger by assuming that he is free from infectious disease.

Suppose the seven-year-old has been exposed to hepatitis C (HCV) but does not yet know he is infected. Though he feels fine and looks healthy, he could still pass the virus on to anyone who comes in contact with his blood, including Nancy.

The point of this example is to show that regardless of how safe the patient looks, he may still be infected with a communicable disease.

**ALERT**

Regardless of the situation, use standard precautions with every patient.

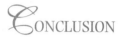 CONCLUSION

By knowing how the disease process works, the employee at risk of occupational exposure can be better protected against exposure to disease.

### CASE STUDY 3.1

Hi. My name is Flo. I am an influenza virus now running rampant in the body of a two-year-old. Would you like to hear the story of how I came to be here?

I'll begin my story with my arrival at ABC Manufacturing. My colleagues and I arrived with the mail carrier who was kind enough to give us a ride. Due to a seemingly innocent sneeze, a few (thousand) of us ended up on the mail for ABC. This is where it gets interesting.

The secretary, Mrs. Howard, carried us to her boss, Mr. West. While reading his mail, Mr. West was paged to the manufacturing area. On the way there, he stopped at the

*(continued)*

water cooler for a drink. A few of my buddies decided to hang around there but I continued on with Mr. West. He is such an hospitable host.

As Mr. West reviewed the order on the foreman's clipboard, I was handed off to Mr. Binden, the foreman. He then transferred me to a work order and passed me on to Mrs. Cooper.

On the way home, Mrs. Cooper stopped at her favorite supermarket to pick up a few things. There she dropped me off on the handle of the shopping cart. Then along came Billy, a curious two-year-old. You know how two-year-olds love to chew on shopping cart handles. Now I'm safe, cozy, and warm with Billy. But not for long...

REFLECT AND CONSIDER

➤ What one simple procedure could have prevented this spread of infection from happening?
➤ Discuss how many opportunities there were to stop the passage of the virus.
➤ List several ways viruses like influenza are spread.

## QUESTIONS FOR DISCUSSION

1. Are all infectious diseases communicable? Explain your answer.
2. Is a person more likely to become infected with HIV through direct or indirect contact? Explain your answer.
3. If you are exposed to a person with HIV today and have a negative blood test tomorrow, are you considered "safe?"

4. Name at least three ways diseases may be transmitted.

5. List at least four causes of infectious disease.

## WORTH THINKING ABOUT

- Which communicable disease(s) are you personally, as a health care provider, the most concerned with?
- What can you do to reduce your opportunity for exposure to communicable disease?

## BIBLIOGRAPHY

National Fire Academy. (1992). *Infection control for emergency response personnel: The supervisor's role.* Emmitsburg, MD: Author.

Neighbors, M., & Tannehill-Jones, R. (2000). *Human diseases.* Albany, NY: Delmar.

Shimeld, L. A., & Rodgers, A. T. (1999). *Essentials of diagnostic microbiology.* Albany, NY: Delmar.

Sugar, A. M., & Lyman, C. A. (1997). *A practical guide to medically important fungi and the diseases they cause.* Philadelphia, PA: Lippincott-Raven.

Thibodeau, G. A., & Patton, K. T. (1999). *Anatomy and physiology.* (4th ed.). St. Louis, MO: Mosby.

United States Fire Administration. (1992). *Guide to developing and managing an emergency service infection control program.*

# $\mathscr{C}$hapter 4
## The Immune System

▼    ▼    ▼    ▼    ▼    ▼    ▼

## $\mathscr{L}$EARNING OBJECTIVES

After completing this chapter, the reader should be able to:

- describe the function and characteristics of the immune system.
- describe the body's defense mechanisms against infections.
- discuss and review anatomy and physiology related to the immune system.
- discuss the process of immune system defenses including humoral and cell-mediated immunity.

## $\mathscr{K}$EY TERMS

- acquired immunity
- active immunity
- antigens
- antibodies
- autoimmune response
- B lymphocytes
- basophils
- cancerous
- cell-mediated immunity
- chemotaxis

- complement proteins
- helper T cells
- humoral immunity
- inflammatory response
- inherited immunity
- integumentary system
- interferon
- killer T cells
- leukocytes
- lymphocytes
- lymphotoxins
- lysozyme
- macrophages
- mast cells
- mitotic
- natural killer cells
- neutrophils
- passive immunity
- phagocytosis
- sebum
- specific immunity
- T lymphocytes
- T suppressor cells
- therapeutic
- tumor

# INTRODUCTION

Every minute of every day, the immune system works to protect the body from pathogens. This chapter is intended to develop a basic understanding of the body's ability to protect itself and what one should expect when this system fails.

# $\mathscr{S}$TRUCTURE OF THE IMMUNE SYSTEM

The immune system is unique in that its components are not contained within one particular organ or organ system. The immune system is comprised of organs and structures from several other body systems, which work together to protect the body from pathogens. Some of the major structures involved in immunity are discussed and illustrated in Figure 4-1.

The tonsils form a protective ring around the upper throat and nose. The palantine tonsils are located on each side of the throat. The lingual tonsils are located near the base of the tongue. The pharyngeal tonsils (sometimes referred to as adenoids) are located near the posterior opening of the nasal cavity. Together, these lymphatic structures protect the entrance of the respiratory system from invading pathogens.

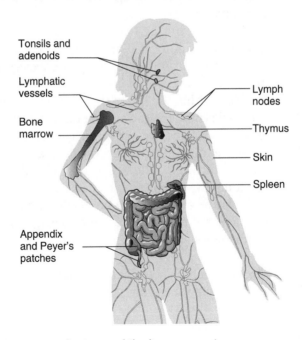

**FIGURE 4-1** Anatomy of the immune system.

Lymph nodes are small oval or bean-shaped structures that range in size from a pin head to a lima bean. Lymph nodes are designed to filter harmful substances including viruses, bacteria, and malignant cells.

Lymphatic vessels are thin-walled tubes that are very similar in structure to veins. These lymphatic vessels carry lymph fluid from the tissues to the larger lymphatic vessels. Like veins, lymphatic vessels utilize valves to prevent the backward flow of lymph fluid.

The thymus is considered the primary organ of the lymphatic system. Located just above (superior to) the heart and just below (inferior to) the thyroid gland, the thymus produces T lymphocytes. As the final site of lymphocyte development before birth, the thymus is relatively large in infants. As we age, the thymus shrinks to the point where little thymus tissue is found in adults.

The spleen is an oval-shaped organ located in the left upper quadrant of the abdomen, just above the left kidney, that serves several functions in the immune system. It is within the spleen that specialized white blood cells called monocytes and lymphocytes complete their development and are activated. The spleen also filters microorganisms and other foreign material from the blood through the process of phagocytosis. Additionally, the spleen serves as a reservoir for blood that may be utilized when needed to destroy worn-out platelets and red blood cells and salvage the reusable components.

The vermiform appendix is a worm-like tube of lymphatic tissue that hangs from the lower portion of the cecum in the large intestine. The appendix serves as what could be described as a breeding ground for intestinal bacteria. While its function is not clear, it is thought that the purpose of the appendix is to harbor nonpathogenic bacteria under normal conditions which helps prevent disease. Peyer's patches are areas of lymphatic tissue located on the walls of the large intestine. They respond to antigens in the intestines by producing plasma cells that secrete antibodies.

The skin is an important part of the immune system. As a natural barrier against foreign pathogens, the skin protects the entire body from invasion. Bone marrow also works with the immune system and is important in the development of erythrocytes and leukocytes. Through the contributions of several body systems and organs working in concert with one another, the body is uniquely able to protect itself from most harmful pathogens.

## FUNCTION OF THE IMMUNE SYSTEM

The immune system protects the body from both external and internal assaults. When harmful microorganisms like viruses, bacteria, or protozoans are introduced into the body, the immune system immediately springs into action to fight against these external assaults. Assaults may also be internal. When abnormal cells replicate and develop **tumors**, the immune system recognizes them as foreign and works to destroy them before they become **cancerous**. Regardless of the source of the pathogen, the immune system constantly works to protect the body from foreign cells.

Sometimes foreign tissues are introduced into the body for **therapeutic** reasons. Organ and tissue transplants are sometimes recognized as foreign by the immune system and are rejected by the body. Occasionally the immune system will erroneously react to any part of the body that it perceives as foreign. This elicits an autoimmune response and may result in illness. Examples of autoimmune disease include lupus, rheumatic fever, multiple sclerosis, and Graves' disease (Figure 4-2).

| Disease | Affected Area |
| --- | --- |
| Crohn's disease | Intestines, the ileum, or the colon |
| Diabetes mellitus, type 1 | Insulin-producing pancreatic cells |
| Graves' disease | Thyroid gland |
| Hashimoto's thyroiditis | Thyroid gland |
| Lupus erythmatosus | Skin and other body systems |
| Myasthenia gravis | Nerve/muscle synapses |
| Multiple sclerosis | Brain and spinal cord |
| Psoriasis | Skin |
| Rheumatoid arthritis | Connective tissue |
| Scleroderma | Skin and other tissues |

FIGURE 4-2 Examples of autoimmune disorders and the body systems they affect.

# THE IMMUNE RESPONSE

When pathogens enter the body, the immune system responds. Immunity typically falls into one of two categories. Specific immunity utilizes lymphocytes (T cells and B cells) to provide protection against specific pathogens. Nonspecific immunity utilizes neutrophils, macrophages, monocytes, and natural killer cells as a more general defense against pathogens. A description of each type of immunity follows.

# $\mathcal{N}$ONSPECIFIC IMMUNITY

The **integumentary system** provides the first line of defense against invasion by providing a structural barrier that prevents pathogens from readily entering the body. The skin also excretes **sebum** and perspiration which mechanically wash pathogens off the skin and chemically attack bacteria. **Lysozyme**, an enzyme that attacks cell walls of gram positive bacteria, causes skin to be acidotic, making it inhospitable to most bacteria. The skin constantly regenerates itself by sloughing off the old layer along with external irritants.

The respiratory system provides protection against inhaled irritants. Coughs and sneezes help remove pathogens from the upper airway, and mucous and cilia within the respiratory tract help to trap and mechanically remove irritants. The structure of the tonsils also protects the entrance of the respiratory system from invading pathogens.

Gastric acids and enzymes also help neutralize pathogens that attack through the gastrointestinal system. The presence of normal bacterial flora may also produce chemicals that inhibit the growth of invading bacteria.

Dangerous pathogens may also be removed from the body via mechanical methods. Pathogens are sloughed off with dead skin cells, vomited from the stomach, flushed from the urinary tract with urine, or caught in respiratory mucous and coughed up. Both the anatomic structure and the mechanical function of the body serve as first line defense against invasion by harmful pathogens.

# INFLAMMATORY RESPONSE

If anatomic barriers like the skin form the first line of protection against pathogens, the inflammatory response provides the second line of protection. The **inflammatory response** utilizes specialized leukocytes called neutrophils and macrophages to find and destroy invading pathogens through a process called phagocytosis.

When an injury or invasion takes place, **leukocytes**, or white blood cells, are summoned to the affected area through a release of leukocyte-attracting chemicals in a process called **chemotaxis**. This results in increased blood flow and vascular permeability in the area, causing the characteristic signs of infection, including hot, swollen, and reddened skin (Figure 4-3).

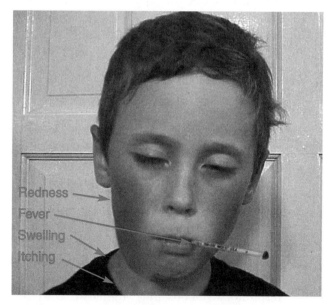

Redness
Fever
Swelling
Itching

**FIGURE 4-3** Health care providers should be alert to the signs and symptoms of infection, including reddened skin, fever, swelling, and itching.

## Phagocytosis

Another part of the inflammatory process is **phagocytosis**. In this process, phagocytes (cells capable of phagocytosis) attack and ingest the invading agent. Phagocytes attack invading pathogens by trapping them with an arm-like projection and encircling them by forming a sac around them. Once enclosed in a sac, the pathogens are chemically destroyed.

Two of the most common phagocytes are **neutrophils** and **macrophages** (Figure 4-4). Neutrophils are the most numerous of the phagocytes. Soon after injury or invasion, neutrophils come out of the capillaries into the affected area where they ingest the microorganisms through phagocytosis and die within one or two days. Due to this short life span, dead neutrophils tend to aggregate and form pus, which is readily absorbed into the surrounding tissues.

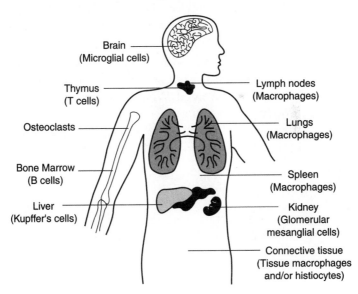

FIGURE 4-4 Cells of the immune system. The immune system is made up of cells from many body systems.

Macrophages migrate out of the bloodstream and grow to several times their original size. They may reside on the surface of mucous membranes for long periods of time. Frequently found in the alveoli, lymph nodes, brain, liver, and spleen, macrophages ingest invading and dead cells. Like neutrophils, dead macrophages tend to collect in the affected area as pus.

### Other Types of Nonspecific Immunity

Other types of nonspecific immunity include the following.

- **natural killer cells**—Natural killer cells are another type of lymphocyte that recognizes and destroys infectious or tumor cells. Natural killer cells do not have to be activated by an external antigen, so they are considered nonspecific.

- **interferon**—Interferon is a protein that defends against viral infections. By inhibiting the ability of a virus to cause a disease, interferon prevents viruses from replicating in cells.

- **complement proteins**—A group of approximately 20 inactivated plasma proteins called complement, circulate in the blood. When activated, complement proteins cause rupture of the cell that triggered them. Complement proteins may be triggered by both specific and nonspecific mechanisms.

## SPECIFIC IMMUNITY

Specific immunity allows the body to defend against specific foreign pathogens within the body. Specific immunity may be either acquired or inherited. **Inherited immunity** is, as the name implies, acquired in utero. **Acquired immunity** may be natural, resulting from nondeliberate exposure to antigens after birth; or artificial, brought about by immunization.

## Active and Passive Immunity

Acquired immunity, whether natural or artificial, may be active or passive. **Active immunity** means that the individual has the ability to produce antibodies to a certain antigen. This type of immunity is longer acting than passive immunity.

**Passive immunity** refers to immunity that is from an outside source or transferred to someone who was not previously immune. Passive immunity provides temporary, but immediate, protection.

## COMPONENTS OF SPECIFIC IMMUNITY

As with nonspecific immunity, several components work together to protect the body from invasion from specific pathogens. Descriptions of some of the more important ones follow.

## Antigens and Antibodies

**Antigens** are chemical markers that identify cells as self (human) or nonself (foreign). When viruses, bacteria, or fungi are recognized as foreign, they are marked as nonself by antigens and subsequently destroyed by the immune system.

**Antibodies** work in a similar fashion, though they are much more specific. Produced in plasma, antibodies are proteins that attach themselves to antigens to mark them for destruction. Each antibody is specific to only one antigen, and the body may produce millions of different antibodies when needed. The five major classes of antibodies follow.

- *Immunoglobulin A (IgA)* is primarily found in the mucous membranes, saliva, and tears. Among other things, it provides passive immunity for breast-fed infants and combines with a protein in the mucosa to defend against invading microorganisms.

- *Immunoglobulin D (IgD)* is found in the B lymphocytes and accounts for less than 1% of antibodies. Its exact function is not known.
- *Immunoglobulin E (IgE)* is found in the mast cells or basophils and accounts for less than 1% of antibodies. It is important to the immediate histamine response in allergic reactions.
- *Immunoglobulin G (IgG)* is the most abundant circulating antibody, and is located in the blood and extracellular fluid. IgG has four subclasses and deals primarily with the secondary immune response. It also has the distinction of being the only immunoglobulin that has the ability to cross the placenta to provide temporary immunity in neonates.
- *Immunoglobulin M (IgM)* is the dominant antibody responsible for the primary immune response. IgM also increases production of IgG in acute infections.

## B Lymphocytes

B lymphocytes (B cells) develop in two stages. Inactive B cells develop by the time an infant reaches a few months of age, and make antibody molecules that attach to the surface of plasma membranes, serving as receptors for specific antigens. After being released from the bone marrow, inactive B cells find their way to the lymph nodes and spleen.

When a B cell comes in contact with the specific antigen that activates it, the antibodies on the B cell's surface bind to the antigen. This triggers a series of mitotic divisions. As this rapid division takes place, the B cell produces a set of clones. Some of these clones form plasma cells, which make and secrete large amounts of antibody. Other clones stay in the lymphatic tissue as memory cells. Should the clone come in contact with the antigen again, memory cells can become plasma cells, which can secrete antibodies, protecting the body from a previously encountered antigen.

## Humoral Immunity

Since B cells do not destroy pathogens directly, but instead produce antibodies that destroy a specific antigen, the process of immunity they produce is called *antibody-mediated immunity*. It is also called **humoral immunity** because it occurs within plasma, which is one of the humors (fluids) in the body.

## T Lymphocytes

**T lymphocytes**, or T cells, attack pathogens directly. The immunity they provide is sometimes referred to as **cell-mediated immunity**. T cells are lymphocytes that develop in the thymus and typically reside in the spleen and lymph nodes. There are three types of T cells.

- **Killer T cells** are able to recognize, bind to, and kill antigens located on the surface of pathogenic cells. By releasing **lymphotoxin**, a powerful poison, T killer cells eliminate pathogens directly.

- **Helper T cells** work with **T suppressor cells** to regulate the function of B cells and other T cells.

## Cell-mediated Immunity

Since T cells directly locate and destroy diseased or pathogenic cells, the type of immunity offered by T cells is referred to as *cell-mediated immunity*. The cells themselves defend the body against dangerous pathogens.

# CONCLUSION

The human body is capable of defending itself against pathogens, both internal and external. The combination of nonspecific and specific immunity assures maximum protection against any pathogen, foreign cell, or cancerous tumor. It is important for health care professionals to understand the fundamentals of the immune system so they can recognize signs that would indicate when the immune system is reacting to a pathogen.

## CASE STUDY 4.1

Hello. I am Luke (a leukocyte), ready to take you for an incredible journey into battle against harmful pathogens. Before we begin, allow me to introduce you to two of my cousins: Mac (a macrophage) and Newt (a neutrophil). Like myself, Mac and Newt are soldiers. Here's how we are activated.

When the enemy attacks (pathogen invasion), we are called to the scene by chemotaxis. You can think of chemotaxis as signals being sent to our troops. We arrive on scene due to increased blood flow and vascular permeability, which causes hot, swollen, red skin. As we arrive, my cousin Newt and his troops come out of the capillaries and ingest the offending microorganism. Unfortunately, neutrophils, which are very numerous, die within one or two days and form pus. Mac, whose troops are fewer in number, will soon arrive and grow to several times his original size as he consumes invading and dead cells. He too will die after his job is done and will accumulate in the affected area as pus.

### REFLECT AND CONSIDER

> Why does someone with an infection have a high white blood cell (WBC) count?

*(continued)*

> ➤ Which is the earlier sign of infection: hot, red skin or the presence of pus?

## QUESTIONS FOR DISCUSSION

1. List and describe some of the key anatomical structures of the immune system?
2. Describe the process of phagocytosis and explain why it results in the production of pus.
3. Which lasts longer, passive or active immunity? Why?
4. Of antigens and antibodies, which are more specific? Why?
5. List several signs and symptoms of infections. Discuss why these signs appear.

## WORTH THINKING ABOUT

• Think of a time when you had an infection. Recall the signs and symptoms you exhibited. What evidence did this give you of your immune system at work?

## BIBLIOGRAPHY

Hegner, B. R., Caldwell, E., & Needham, J. F. (1999). *Nursing assistant: A nursing process approach.* (8th ed.). Albany, NY: Delmar.

Neighbors, M., & Tannehill-Jones, R. (2000). *Human diseases.* Albany, NY: Delmar.

Smith, J. (1995). *Immunology: The clinical laboratory manual series.* Albany, NY: Delmar.

Thibodeau, G. A., & Patton, K. T. (1999). *Anatomy and physiology.* (4th ed.). St. Louis, MO: Mosby.

Van Wynsberghe, D., Noback, C. R., & Carola, R. (1995). *Human anatomy and physiology.* (3rd ed.). New York, NY: McGraw-Hill.

# Chapter 5
## Diseases of Concern

▼   ▼   ▼   ▼   ▼   ▼   ▼

## LEARNING OBJECTIVES

After completing this chapter, the reader should be able to:

- understand which diseases health care providers are most susceptible to.
- know general patient management and protective measures for each disease.
- be aware of some common infectious diseases and have learned the causative agent(s), route(s) of transmission, and susceptibility of each of the following:
  - acquired immunodeficiency syndrome (AIDS)
  - amebiasis
  - anthrax
  - botulism
  - chlamydia
  - chickenpox
  - cryptosporidosis
  - cytomegalovirus
  - *escherichia coli*
  - gonorrhea
  - Hantavirus Pulmonary Syndrome
  - hepatitis A
  - hepatitis B
  - hepatitis C
  - hepatitis non-ABC

- herpes simplex 1
- herpes simplex 2
- influenza
- legionellosis
- lice
- listeriosis
- lyme disease
- measles
- meningococcal meningitis
- mononucleosis
- mumps
- pertussis
- pneumonia
- rabies
- Rocky Mountain Spotted Fever
- rubella
- salmonellosis
- scabies
- shigellosis
- syphilis
- tetanus
- tuberculosis

# KEY TERMS

NOTE:  Since each of the infectious diseases discussed in this chapter are defined and explained within this chapter, they are not included in the key terms section of this chapter. They are, however, defined in the glossary.

- adsorb
- antiviral
- aphasia
- asymptomatic

- attenuated
- Bell's Palsy
- causative agent
- chancre
- congenital rubella syndrome (CRS)
- conjunctivitis
- debridement
- disseminated intravascular coagulation (DIC)
- dormant
- dysuria
- encephalitis
- enteric
- enterohemorrhagic
- environmentally resistant
- epididymitis
- exudates
- Gullain-Barre Syndrome
- hemolytic uremic syndrome
- Koplik's spots
- lacrimation
- lesion
- Mantoux test
- mite
- myalgia
- myoclomus
- necrosis
- nonsteroidal anti-inflammatory drugs (NSAIDS)
- nuchal rigidity
- nymph
- oocyst
- paresthesia
- pathogenic
- pediculicide

- pelvic inflammatory disease (PID)
- peripheral neuropathy
- petechial rash
- photophobia
- prodromal
- prostatitis
- purulent
- replicate
- septic arthritis
- susceptible
- systemic bacteremia
- thrombocytopaenia
- urethral strictures

# INTRODUCTION

This chapter is a quick reference for the health care provider. The information contained within may be considered an overview of the various diseases covered. The reader is encouraged to seek additional resources about a variety of infectious diseases not listed here.

Each disease listed includes information on the causative agent, or what bacteria, virus, fungus, protozoa, or rickettsia causes the disease. Next, the body systems typically affected by the disease is shown, followed by a brief description of who, if anyone, is most susceptible to this particular disease. Routes of transmission are discussed, as are common signs and symptoms, and patient management procedures. Next, protective measures that should be taken by the health care provider are listed followed by the availability of a vaccine for the disease. Finally, the incubation period for the disease is listed and a section labeled "HCP Tips" lists some things a health care provider may need to know about this disease.

Icons shown in Figure 5-1 are used to facilitate ease of use.

Health care provider alert          Vaccine available

FIGURE 5-1 These icons will be utilized throughout this chapter as a quick reference for the reader.

# ACQUIRED IMMUNODEFICIENCY SYNDROME (AIDS)

| | |
|---|---|
| **Causative Agent** | AIDS is caused by the human immuno-deficiency virus (HIV), specifically HIV 1 and HIV 2. HIV 1 is far more pathogenic than HIV 2. Most known cases are HIV 1 Group M. |
| **Body Systems Affected** | HIV primarily affects the immune system and may also affect the nervous, respiratory, and integumentary systems. |
| **Susceptibility** | Persons with pre-existing sexually transmitted diseases (STDs), those who have unprotected sex with multiple partners, and intravenous drug users who share needles are at increased risk of contracting the HIV virus. |
| **Routes of Transmission** | HIV may be transmitted through unprotected sexual contact, sharing intravenous needles, and needlesticks. |
| **Signs and Symptoms** | Signs and symptoms vary but may include fatigue, night sweats, fever, diarrhea, swollen lymph nodes, skin lesions (Figure 5-2), and unexplained weight loss. The HIV-infected patient may remain asymptomatic for months or years. |

**Patient Management**   Care is primarily supportive. Treat signs and symptoms.

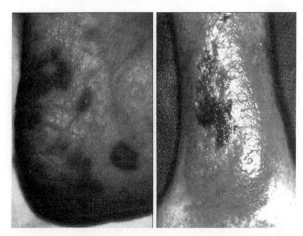

FIGURE 5-2 Kaposi's sarcoma. This cancer of the blood vessels, which causes reddish-purple skin lesions, may be found in HIV patients.

**Protective Measures**   Body Substance Isolation (BSI) is indicated. Be especially careful when handling any blood or blood-containing body fluids.

**Immunizations**   There is no vaccine available for HIV or AIDS at this time.

**Incubation Period**   The incubation period for HIV may be up to ten years.

**Health Care Providers**   Though occupational exposure to HIV is rare, health care providers should isolate themselves from contact with blood or blood-containing body fluids. Since HIV does not survive long outside the human body, greatest risk for transmission to health care providers is through a needle-stick.

# Amebiasis

| | |
|---|---|
| **Causative Agent** | Amebiasis is caused by a microscopic parasite called *Entamoeba histolytica*. |
| **Body Systems Affected** | This parasitic disease affects the gastrointestinal system. |
| **Susceptibility** | Susceptibility is general though those who visit tropical climates are more likely to be exposed. |
| **Routes of Transmission** | Transmission can be person-to-person through contact with fecal material, by drinking contaminated water, or eating contaminated food. |
| **Signs and Symptoms** | Most experience few, if any symptoms. Symptoms, if they appear, are typically mild and may include nausea, diarrhea, and abdominal pain. |
| **Patient Management** | Management is generally supportive. Antibiotics and intravenous fluid therapy may be indicated. |
| **Protective Measures** | As with any patient, personal protective equipment (PPE) should be utilized and hand washing should be thorough. |
| **Immunizations** | There is no immunization for amebiasis at this time. |
| **Incubation Period** | Incubation period for amebiasis may be from a few days to a few months. Typical incubation period is 2–4 weeks. |
| **Health Care Providers** | Health care providers should use typical protective measures and avoid contact with any fecal material. |

# $\mathcal{A}$NTHRAX (WOOLSORTERS' DISEASE)

**Causative Agent**

Anthrax is a bacterial disease that can infect any warm-blooded animal, including humans.

**Body Systems Affected**

Anthrax affects the integumentary, lymphatic, and respiratory systems.

**Susceptibility**

Though anthrax may be used as a biological weapon, it is typically considered an occupational disease for those who have exposure to dead animals and animal products.

**Routes of Transmission**

Anthrax may be spread by handling contaminated wool or hair or by eating undercooked meat from diseased animals. Anthrax may also live in the soil and may be transmitted by inhaling contaminated soil particles.

**Signs and Symptoms**

Signs and symptoms vary with the type of exposure. Exposure to the skin can cause boil-like lesions. Inhalation of anthrax may cause symptoms that resemble a cold and may progress to respiratory distress or failure.

**Patient Management**

Care is supportive with emphasis on ventilatory support. Penicillin or tetracycline may he helpful.

**Protective Measures**

There are no reported cases of anthrax being spread person-to-person. However, opportunity for exposure to the health care provider exists when the source of the disease may be present. Respiratory protection is indicated as is standard BSI.

**Immunizations**

There is a vaccine for anthrax which is recommended for those who work in occupations with potential for exposure.

**Incubation Period**   Incubation period of anthrax is usually less than seven days.

**Health Care Providers**   Health care providers should be cautious on two fronts. When treating persons with potential occupational exposure to anthrax, health care providers should take care to barrier themselves from any potentially contaminated materials. Care should also be taken to decontaminate the patient.

In today's world, health care providers should also be aware of the potential for use of anthrax as a biological weapon. Rapid recognition of the signs and symptoms of anthrax in a multiple-patient situation coupled with the everyday practice of careful body substance isolation could help avert a major incident.

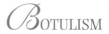

# BOTULISM

**Causative Agent**   Botulism is a type of food poisoning caused by a toxin produced by the *Clostridium botulinum* bacteria.

**Body Systems Affected**   Botulism affects the nervous system.

**Susceptibility**   Susceptibility for botulism is general.

**Routes of Transmission**   Transmission of botulism is through ingestion of undercooked food contaminated with the *Clostridium botulinum* bacteria. There is no evidence of person-to-person transmission of botulism. Infants are sometimes infected through the ingestion of contaminated honey.

| | |
|---|---|
| **Signs and Symptoms** | Symptoms of botulism may include weakness, poor reflexes, blurred or double vision, and difficulty swallowing. Symptoms of infant botulism may include visual disturbances, poor feeding, and difficulty breathing. |
| **Patient Management** | Treatment for botulism is generally supportive. An antitoxin may be given in certain cases of foodborne botulism but not with infant botulism. |
| **Protective Measures** | Since botulism is not spread person-to-person, standard precautions should be adequate protection. |
| **Immunizations** | There is no vaccine for botulism at this time. |
| **Incubation Period** | The incubation period for botulism may be between 12 hours and several days. The appearance of symptoms within 36 hours is not uncommon. |
| **Health Care Providers** | Since botulism is foodborne, health care providers should take care to properly cook and reheat food. Bulging cans should not be opened and honey should not be given to infants (under one year). |

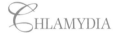HLAMYDIA

| | |
|---|---|
| **Causative Agent** | *Chlamydia trachomatis* is the causative agent for chlamydia. |
| **Body Systems Affected** | *Chlamydia* affects the eyes, genitals, and respiratory system. |
| **Susceptibility** | Susceptibility is general. It is estimated that 25% of men may be carriers. Unlike some other diseases, it appears there is no acquired immunity for *chlamydia* after infection. |

| | |
|---|---|
| **Routes of Transmission** | *Chlamydia* is typically considered a sexually transmitted disease though it may be transmitted by sharing contaminated clothing or towels. Infected eye secretions may be transmitted hand-to-hand. |
| **Signs and Symptoms** | Common signs and symptoms include **conjuctivitis, dysuria** and **purulent** urinary discharge. |
| **Patient Management** | Patient care is supportive. Antibiotics may be prescribed. |
| **Protective Measures** | Body substance isolation and diligent hand washing should be practiced. |
| **Immunizations** | No immunization is available at this time. |
| **Incubation Period** | Incubation period is one week to one month. |
| **Health Care Providers** | Health care providers should take care in handling contaminated clothing or linens. All contaminated linen should be placed in a biohazard bag and treated as infectious. As always, good hand washing is essential. |

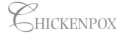

# CHICKENPOX

| | |
|---|---|
| **Causative Agent** | Chickenpox is caused by the varicella-zoster virus. |
| **Body Systems Affected** | The integumentary system is the primary body system affected. |
| **Susceptibility** | Susceptibility is general. |
| **Routes of Transmission** | Chickenpox is considered an airborne transmitted disease though it may be transmitted by contact with items contaminated with discharges from skin lesions of an infected person. |

**Signs and Symptoms**      A rash, primarily on the trunk, begins as small red spots that become blisters (Figure 5-3). Once these blisters collapse, they dry into scabs. Patients also experience respiratory symptoms, generalized weakness, and low-grade fever.

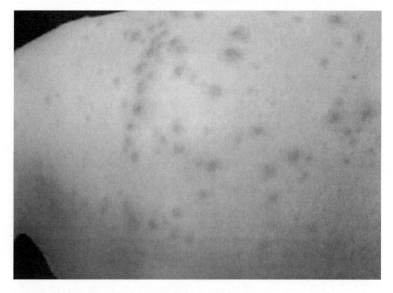

FIGURE 5-3 Chicken pox. (Photo courtesy of the Centers for Disease Control and Prevention.)

**Patient Management**      Care is primarily supportive. **Antiviral** drugs may be helpful.

**Protective Measures**      Persons with chickenpox should avoid public places until all **lesions** are crusted and dry. Health care providers should use BSI, take care in handling soiled linen, and wash hands thoroughly after patient contact.

**Immunizations**      A vaccine is available and recommended for unvaccinated or non-immune health

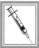

care providers. The vaccine should not be given to pregnant women or those with depressed immune systems.

**Incubation Period**

Incubation period may be between 7 and 21 days, though it is typically 14–17 days.

**Health Care Providers**

Health care providers who can not prove immunity to chicken pox should take the live, attenuated varicella vaccine. While there is some controversy surrounding how immunity should be proved, the CDC suggests that confirmation by a parent or other responsible adult of someone having chicken pox during childhood should be adequate to suggest immunity.

BSI should be used and extreme care should be taken in handling soiled linens. All contaminated linens should be placed in a biohazard bag.

# CRYPTOSPORIDIOSIS

**Causative Agent**

The causative agent of cryptosporidiosis is cryptosporidium, a single-celled parasitic protozoan which lives in the intestines of people and animals. The dormant (inactive) form is oocyst which is excreted from the feces of infected humans and animals. Oocyst is environmentally resistant and can survive outside of the body for long periods of time.

**Body Systems Affected**

The primary body system affected by cryptosporidiosis is the gastrointestinal (GI) system.

**Susceptibility**

Susceptibility is general, though those with weakened immune systems tend to have more severe symptoms. Anyone who consumes contaminated food or water or is exposed to the fecal material of an infected person may be at risk. Entire municipal water systems have been affected. Outbreaks of Cryptosporidiosis have been documented in Carrollton, Georgia and Milwaukee, Wisconsin. In Milwaukee, an estimated 400,000 people became ill during a single outbreak. Additional outbreaks have been documented at day care centers.

**Routes of Transmission**   This disease is basically waterborne though it may be transmitted person-to-person through exposure to the feces of an infected person.

**Signs and Symptoms**   Signs and symptoms include watery diarrhea, abdominal cramps, fever, dehydration, weight loss, and nausea.

**Patient Management**   Management is supportive. Persons who are dehydrated or susceptible to dehydration may need intravenous fluid therapy.

**Protective Measures**   Body substance isolation (BSI) measures should be utilized with all patients. Specifically, **enteric** precautions should be taken and hand washing should be meticulous.

**Immunizations**   There is no immunization available at this time.

**Incubation Period**   Incubation period typically is between 2–10 days though the average is seven days.

**Health Care Providers**   Health care providers should remember that oocysts are not killed with typical disinfectants. Heat of 160°F is necessary to kill the protozoa. Good hand washing,

BSI, and care in handling soiled linens and equipment should be taken.

# CYTOMEGALOVIRUS (CMV)

**Causative Agent**

The causative agent of CMV is cytomegalovirus, a member of the herpesvirus group. Though very common, CMV rarely causes illness and often goes undetected.

**Body Systems Affected**

In the average person, CMV will cause no significant effects. However, in the immunocompromised patient, the eyes may be affected. Persons with AIDS may experience retinal infections which could lead to blindness.

**Susceptibility**

Susceptibility is general in that anyone may become infected. However, CMV infection is more likely in developing countries and in areas with low socioeconomic conditions. Risks are also greater for unborn babies and newborns as well as for those who are immunocompromised.

**Routes of Transmission**

CMV infection is typically transmitted through urine, saliva, blood, semen, tears, or breast milk of an infected person. Person-to-person transmission usually takes place when infected body fluid comes in contact with the hands and the hands spread the infection to the mouth or nose. It can also be sexually transmitted.

**Signs and Symptoms**

Though CMV seldom causes illness, when signs and symptoms occur they may appear similar to those seen with infectious mononucleosis. Signs like fatigue, malaise, fever, chills, and muscle aches may be expected. Immunocompromised persons and those who have received organ transplants may experience more dangerous symptoms including infections of the retina and blindness.

**Patient Management**

Most persons with CMV do not require treatment. Treatment, when indicated, is supportive. Pharmacological therapy using ganciclovir and foscarnet may be helpful in the immunocompromised patient, though they are not recommended for the otherwise healthy patient due to the sometimes severe side effects they may cause.

**Protective Measures**

As with any patient, BSI and good hand washing should be observed. Use care when handling contaminated linens, equipment, and personal effects of infected patients as the virus may be active on these surfaces.

**Immunizations**

An immunization for CMV is in the early stages of development, but is not yet available.

**Incubation Period**

The typical incubation period is 20–60 days though it may be shorter in the immunocompromised patient.

**Health Care Providers**

Health care providers should observe BSI and good hand washing. Limit exposure to personal items and place exposed linens in a biohazard bag. Decontaminate all affected equipment.

# &SCHERICHIA COLI (E. COLI)

| | |
|---|---|
| **Causative Agent** | *Escherichia coli* are bacteria normally found in the intestines of humans and animals. Most strains of *E. coli* are harmless, but *E. coli* 0157:H7, a member of the **enterohemorrhagic** group, can cause severe illness. |
| **Body Systems Affected** | *E. coli* 0157:H7 affects the gastrointestinal system and the kidneys. |
| **Susceptibility** | Susceptibility for *E. coli* is general. |
| **Routes of Transmission** | Transmission is primarily foodborne, caused by eating undercooked meat containing the bacteria. However, person-to-person transmission can take place when bacteria from diarrheal stools of infected persons are spread through inadequate hygiene and/or hand washing. |
| **Signs and Symptoms** | The most common complaints are diarrhea (sometimes bloody), and abdominal cramps which last 5–10 days. In severe cases, the infection can cause **hemolytic uremic syndrome**, in which red blood cells are destroyed and kidneys eventually fail. |
| **Patient Management** | Care is supportive and may include fluid replacement to combat dehydration. |
| **Protective Measures** | BSI, good hand washing, and specifically, enteric precautions must be taken. |
| **Immunizations** | There is no vaccination for *E. coli* at this time. |
| **Incubation Period** | Symptoms usually appear in about three days, though the range may be between 1–9 days. |

**Health Care Providers**  Health care providers should observe BSI and good hand washing practices. Avoid handling fecal material and place all contaminated materials in biohazard bags.

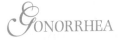

# Gonorrhea

**Causative Agent**  *Neisseria gonorrhea* is the causative agent for gonorrhea.

**Body Systems Affected**  Gonorrhea typically affects genital organs and associated structures.

**Susceptibility**  Susceptibility is general but targeted to those who have unprotected sexual intercourse with infected persons. After exposure, antibodies develop, but only for the specific strain of gonorrhea involved. Those who have been previously exposed may be at greater risk for infection by another strain.

**Routes of Transmission**  Transmission is through direct contact with exudates of mucous membranes and almost always occurs through unprotected sexual intercourse.

**Signs and Symptoms**  Males typically complain of an inflammation of the urethra with associated dysuria and purulent urinary discharge. If untreated, this can progress to epididymitis, prostatitis, and urethral strictures.

Females typically complain of dysuria with a purulent vaginal discharge. Untreated, gonorrhea may progress to pelvic inflammatory disease (PID), causing lower abdominal pain, fever, and abnormal menstrual bleeding. Menstruation gives bacteria the opportunity to spread from the cervix to the upper genital tract and causes 50% of PID cases occurring within one week of the onset of menstruation. Gonorrhea puts females at increased risk of ectopic pregnancy; sterility; and abscesses of the ovaries, fallopian tubes, and other reproductive structures. In rare cases, a **systemic bacteremia** may occur, causing **septic arthritis** with swelling of the joints accompanied by fever and pain. If left untreated, progressive deterioration of the joints may occur.

**Patient Management**

Initial treatment is supportive. Antibiotics may be indicated.

**Protective Measures**

BSI and good hand washing are essential. Place affected linens in biohazard bags and decontaminate exposed equipment.

**Immunizations**

There is no vaccine available for gonorrhea at this time.

**Incubation Period**

Average incubation period is 3–7 days though it may range from a low of 2 days to a high of 30 days.

**Health Care Providers**

Health care providers should use extreme caution when handling soiled linen and should consider any body fluid as potentially infectious.

# HANTAVIRUS PULMONARY SYNDROME

**Causative Agent**

Hantavirus is the causative agent.

**Body Systems Affected**

Hantavirus pulmonary syndrome, as its name suggests, eventually affects the respiratory system. The musculoskeletal system may also be affected.

| | |
|---|---|
| **Susceptibility** | Susceptibility is general. Persons who live or work in areas where rodents or rodent droppings may be found are more likely to be exposed. |
| **Routes of Transmission** | It is thought that Hantavirus is spread when humans inhale microscopic particles that contain rodent droppings or urine. |
| **Signs and Symptoms** | Persons with Hantavirus pulmonary syndrome may be expected to complain of muscle aches, headaches, and coughs. A high fever may also occur. After a few days the patient may develop respiratory symptoms, which may develop into pulmonary edema and eventually, respiratory failure. |
| **Patient Management** | Management is primarily supportive. Some physicians have used ribavarin in an attempt to treat the disease. |
| **Protective Measures** | This disease is not considered person-to-person transmissible, so nothing more than standard precautions are indicated when caring for a patient with Hantavirus pulmonary syndrome. However, when working in rodent-infested areas, the health care provider should wear eye and respiratory protection and should avoid contact with rodents or their droppings. |
| **Immunizations** | There is no vaccine for Hantavirus pulmonary syndrome at this time. |
| **Incubation Period** | The incubation period may range from a few days to six weeks. Typical incubation period is 1–2 weeks. |
| **Health Care Providers** | Health care providers should use caution any time they are exposed to an area infested by rodents. Masks, eye protection, and gloves are indicated to barrier oneself from the disease-causing agent. |

# *H*EPATITIS A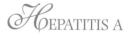

**Causative Agent**

Hepatitis A is caused by the hepatitis A virus.

**Body Systems Affected**

All forms of hepatitis affect the liver.

**Susceptibility**

Susceptibility is general in that there is no clearly defined population at increased risk of hepatitis A. However, those with potential for exposure to fecal material are more likely to be exposed.

**Routes of Transmission**

Hepatitis A may be transmitted person-to-person through the fecal-oral route. Since hepatitis A can survive on unwashed hands for up to four hours, day care workers should be careful to observe good hand washing practices. It may also be transmitted through contaminated water or food, and in some cases may be transmitted through sexual or household contact.

**Signs and Symptoms**

Many infected persons are asymptomatic. Those who experience symptoms may complain of right upper quadrant abdominal pain, anorexia, nausea, fever, and weakness. Symptoms are typically mild in severity and last no more than six weeks.

**Patient Management**

Care is supportive with emphasis on treating the symptoms.

**Protective Measures**

BSI and good hand washing should be the rule with all patients. Special care should be taken to isolate the caregiver from contact with fecal material.

**Immunizations**

An inactivated hepatitis A vaccine is available. The CDC suggests that immunization against hepatitis A may be indicated for health care workers.

| | |
|---|---|
| **Incubation Period** | Incubation period is typically 2–6 weeks. |
| **Health Care Providers** | Health care providers should take care to isolate themselves from fecal material through BSI and should practice good hand washing habits. Immunization against hepatitis A should be considered. |

# 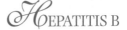 HEPATITIS B

| | |
|---|---|
| **Causative Agent** | Hepatitis B virus is the causative agent. |
| **Body Systems Affected** | Hepatitis B affects the liver and may cause **necrosis**. |
| **Susceptibility** | Susceptibility is general, though those with exposure to infected blood or blood-containing body fluids are at greater risk. |
| **Routes of Transmission** | Blood, semen, vaginal fluids, and saliva may all be considered infectious. Hepatitis B may be transmitted through exposure to blood and blood-containing body fluid through occupational exposure, sexual contact, or contact with contaminated needles. |
| **Signs and Symptoms** | Persons infected with hepatitis B typically complain of cold and flu-like symptoms including fever, joint pain, general weakness, anorexia, and nausea and vomiting. Since the disease affects the liver, jaundice may occur. |
| **Patient Management** | Care for the patient with hepatitis B is primarily supportive. |
| **Protective Measures** | BSI is essential, as is effective hand washing. |
| **Immunizations**  | Recombinant vaccines (Recombivax HB and Engerix B) are available and given in a series of three intramuscular injections. |

The first dose is given, followed in one month by a second dose. The third and final dose is given six months after the initial dose. For more information on the hepatitis B vaccine, see Chapter 6.

**Incubation Period**

The incubation period for hepatitis B is typically 1–6 months though it may be as long as 200 days.

**Health Care Providers**

Hepatitis B is environmentally resistant, which means the virus can survive outside the body for long periods of time. Because of this, health care providers should use extreme caution when dealing with any blood or blood-containing body fluid. Body substance isolation and good hand washing techniques are essential as are proper disposal of contaminated linens, equipment, and supplies. Experts tell us that the environmental resistance of hepatitis B makes it 200 times easier to become infected with HBV than with HIV.

# HEPATITIS C

**Causative Agent**

The causative agent is the hepatitis C virus.

**Body Systems Affected**

Hepatitis C primarily affects the liver.

**Susceptibility**

Susceptibility to hepatitic C virus is greater for health care providers than for the general population. When exposed to blood containing the virus, health care providers experience a 2.7–10% probability of contracting the infection. Probability of contracting the disease through household or sexual contact is lower.

Hepatitis C is not known to be transmitted through contaminated food or water.

**Routes of Transmission**  Hepatitis C is transmitted through blood or blood-containing body fluid. Typical routes of transmission are through needlesticks or accidental exposure to blood or blood-containing body fluids. Exposure may be through splashes into the mucous membranes around the eyes, nose, or mouth or through blood coming in contact with non-intact skin.

**Signs and Symptoms**  When symptoms are present, they typically mimic the symptoms of the flu. Often there are no symptoms so by the time a person finds out he/she has hepatitis C, there may already be serious liver damage.

**Patient Management**  Treatment is supportive, though an extensive regimen of pharmacologic therapy is available. This 48-week course of antiviral drugs suppresses the virus in 41% of those who test positive for the disease.

**Protective Measures**  BSI and effective hand washing are essential.

**Immunizations**  Though a vaccine is currently under development, no immunization is currently available.

**Incubation Period**  Incubation period may range between 2–26 weeks, though the average incubation period is 6–8 weeks.

**Health Care Providers**

Health care providers who are expected to have occupational exposure to blood and other potentially infectious material are at risk for becoming infected with the hepatitis C virus. Thousands of health care providers who did not use personal protective equipment and BSI in the 1970s and

1980s have contracted the disease. Since many infected persons are asymptomatic, severe liver damage can occur before learning of the infection.

# $\mathcal{H}$EPATITIS NON-ABC

**Causative Agent**

The primary viruses responsible for non-ABC hepatitis include hepatitis D (delta) virus; hepatitis E, which is similar to hepatitis A; and hepatitis G, which is a newly-identified virus.

**Body Systems Affected**

As with all strains of hepatitis, non-ABC hepatitis viruses affect the liver.

**Susceptibility**

Susceptibility is general, though it should be noted that the hepatitis D virus requires the presence of hepatitis B to **replicate**. When the hepatitis D virus becomes active in people infected with hepatitis B, the resulting disease becomes extremely **pathogenic**.

**Routes of Transmission**

Hepatitis D and G are bloodborne, while hepatitis E is transmitted through exposure to infected fecal matter.

**Signs and Symptoms**

The onset of hepatitis D is abrupt, with signs and symptoms mimicking the hepatitis B virus. It is always associated with, and often mistaken for, hepatitis B. Many patients with hepatitis E are asymptomatic. Symptoms, when they occur, include nausea, fever, abdominal pain, and generalized weakness.

**Patient Management**

Care is supportive.

**Protective Measures**

BSI and effective hand washing are essential.

| | |
|---|---|
| Immunizations | Hepatitis B vaccine can indirectly prevent hepatitis D but has no effect on hepatitis E. Immunity to hepatitis B equates to immunity to hepatitis D. |
| Incubation Period | The incubation period of hepatitis D is 21–90 days. Hepatitis E incubation period may range from 15–60 days, though 40 days is the average. The incubation period of hepatitis G is not yet known. |
| Health Care Providers | Though there is still much to be learned about hepatitis non-ABC, health care providers should take appropriate BSI precautions with all patients and stay abreast of emerging developments in these diseases. |

# $\mathscr{H}$ERPES SIMPLEX 1

| | |
|---|---|
| Causative Agent | Herpes simplex 1 is caused by the herpes simplex virus 1 (HSV 1). |
| Body Systems Affected | Herpes simplex 1 affects the oropharnyx, face, lips, skin, fingers, toes, and, in infants, the central nervous system. |
| Susceptibility | Susceptibility is general. |
| Routes of Transmission | Herpes simplex virus is typically transmitted through saliva and infection on the hands. |
| Signs and Symptoms | Patients will likely experience cold sores and fever blisters, generally found on the lips, face, conjuctiva, or oropharnyx. |
| Patient Management | Care is supportive. Pharmacological therapy with acyclovir (Zovirax) is available. |
| Protective Measures | BSI, including mask and gloves, is recommended. |

| Immunizations | No vaccine is available at this time. |
| Incubation Period | The incubation period of herpes simplex 1 is not yet known. |
| Health Care Providers | Since lesions are highly contagious, health care providers should take care to observe BSI including use of masks and gloves. |

# HERPES SIMPLEX TYPE 2 (GENITAL HERPES)

| Causative Agent | Herpes simplex virus type 2 (HSV2) is the causative agent for genital herpes. |
| Body Systems Affected | Body regions affected include those regions associated with intimate sexual contact. |
| Susceptibility | Susceptibility is general. |
| Routes of Transmission | Transmission is through sexual intercourse. |
| Signs and Symptoms | Males complain of lesions of the penis, anus, rectum, and/or mouth depending on the sexual practices of the affected person. |
| | Females are sometimes asymptomatic but may complain of lesions on the anus, rectum, vulva, cervix, or mouth depending on the sexual practices of the affected person. Recurrences generally affect the buttocks, legs, perineal skin, and vulva. |
| Patient Management | Care is supportive. Pharmacological therapy with acyclovir (Zovirax) may be helpful. |
| Protective Measures | BSI is recommended and especially important when handling affected linen and supplies. |

| | |
|---|---|
| **Immunizations** | There is no vaccine for genital herpes at this time. |
| **Incubation Period** | The incubation period for herpes simplex 2 is not yet known. |
| **Health Care Providers** | Health care providers should use extreme caution when handling linen or equipment exposed to the affected area(s). BSI, used consistently, and effective hand washing are the best lines of defense for the health care provider. |

# ℐNFLUENZA

| | |
|---|---|
| **Causative Agent** | Influenza results from Influenza virus types A, B, and C. |
| **Body Systems Affected** | Influenza primarily affects the respiratory system. |
| **Susceptibility** | Susceptibility is general. Persons at greatest risk of influenza are those who have the greatest opportunity for exposure and those who have weakened immune systems. |
| **Routes of Transmission** | Influenza is spread by inhaling droplets from a sneeze or cough, or by touching an object exposed to the influenza virus then touching the mouth, nose, or mucous membranes around the eyes. |
| **Signs and Symptoms** | Symptoms include fever, chills, headache, muscle aches, sore throat, and a severe and protracted cough. |
| **Patient Management** | Patient care is supportive and is aimed at making the symptoms more tolerable. |
| **Protective Measures** | BSI precautions should be taken. When in close contact with the patient and when |

not otherwise contraindicated, the patient, as well as the caregiver, should wear a mask.

**Immunizations**

Immunizations are widely available and are recommended for persons over 65 years of age, residents of long term care facilities, persons with chronic medical conditions, persons with serious health conditions, anyone with a weakened immune system, and health care providers. Protection develops approximately two weeks after vaccination and lasts approximately one year.

**Incubation Period**

Incubation period is typically 1–3 days.

**Health Care Providers**

Since health care providers are likely to come in contact with persons who have the influenza virus, they should consider taking the influenza vaccine and should always observe BSI and wash their hands after contact with each patient.

# _L_EGIONELLOSIS

**Causative Agent**

Legionellosis is caused by the *Legionella pneumophilia*. This particular bacteria was renamed after an outbreak among people attending an American Legion convention in 1976.

**Body Systems Affected**

Since legionellosis typically causes a bacterial pneumonia, the respiratory system is the primary system affected.

**Susceptibility**

Though susceptibility is general, the disease most often affects middle-aged or older men, especially those who drink

| | alcohol or smoke heavily, and persons with pre-existing medical conditions. |
|---|---|
| **Routes of Transmission** | It is thought that legionellosis is spread through the air from a soil or water source. There is no evidence that person-to-person exposure occurs. |
| **Signs and Symptoms** | Patients typically exhibit flu-like symptoms including muscle aches, headache, fever, chills, and diarrhea. |
| **Patient Management** | Immediate care is supportive. Antibiotics may be helpful in treating the disease. |
| **Protective Measures** | Since there is no evidence to support the belief that legionellosis can be spread person-to-person, standard precautions are all that is recommended. *Legionella* may be found in institutional water systems, ponds and creeks, and in the water in air conditioning units. |
| **Immunizations** | There is currently no vaccine for legionellosis. |
| **Incubation Period** | Signs and symptoms typically occur within five to six days, though a range of 2–10 days has been recorded. |
| **Health Care Providers** | Since legionellosis is not transmitted person-to-person, routine BSI should be adequate protection. This disease occurs sporadically and in outbreaks. |

## $\mathcal{L}$ICE (PEDICULOSIS AND PHTHIRIASIS)

| | |
|---|---|
| **Causative Agent** | Three types of lice are discussed here: *Pediculosis humanus capitis* (head louse), *Pediculosis humanus corporis* (body louse), and *Phthirus pubis* (crab louse). |

| | |
|---|---|
| **Body Systems Affected** | All three types of lice affect the skin and hair (Figure 5-4). |
| **Susceptibility** | Susceptibility is general. |
| **Routes of Transmission** | Head lice are spread through direct contact with an infested person and/or objects used by him or her. Body lice may be spread through indirect contact with personal belongings of an infested person, especially shared clothing and headwear. Crab lice are spread through sexual contact. |

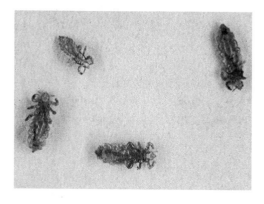

FIGURE 5-4  Detail of head lice.

| | |
|---|---|
| **Signs and Symptoms** | The primary symptom is itching at the affected area. Head lice typically infest head and facial hair. Body lice typically infest the inner seams of clothing. Crab lice infest the genital area. |
| **Patient Management** | A **pediculicide** should be used at time of diagnosis and repeated seven days later. Careful attention to removing all nits, or |

eggs attached to the hair shaft, is necessary. Vinegar and water may be used to loosen the nits prior to combing with a specialized, fine-toothed comb called a delousing comb.

**Protective Measures**    BSI and thorough hand washing should be utilized. Linen should be bagged and the area sprayed with an insecticide known to be effective for lice and mites. Care should be taken to clean and remove insecticide residues.

**Immunizations**    There is no vaccine for lice at this time.

**Incubation Period**    An adult louse can produce approximately six eggs every 24 hours. Eggs hatch in 7–10 days. Depending on the temperature, the **nymph** stage lasts 7–13 days. The egg-to-egg cycle lasts about three weeks.

**Health Care Providers**    Health care providers should remain alert to the presence of lice on their patients and check themselves thoroughly after contact with those known or believed to be infested with lice. Careful attention to checking for lice and/or nits is suggested.

# $\mathcal{L}$ISTERIOSIS

**Causative Agent**    Listeriosis is a bacterial infection caused by the *Listeria* bacteria. One of the most common types is *Listeria monocytogenes*. One trait of *listeria monocytogenes* is that it will grow at refrigeration temperatures and will survive pasteurization and heat treatment. Freezing has little effect on the bacteria. *Listeria monocytogenes* is often found in soil and water.

| | |
|---|---|
| Body Systems Affected | Listeriosis can cause flu-like symptoms and affect the gastrointestinal and nervous systems. |
| Susceptibility | People with weakened immune systems, pregnant women, elderly persons, and those with pre-existing medical conditions are more susceptible to listeriosis than the general population. |
| Routes of Transmission | Listeriosis is typically transmitted through contaminated food, but may be transmitted to a fetus through the placenta of an infected pregnant woman. |
| Signs and Symptoms | Patients with listeriosis experience flu-like symptoms including fever, chills, nausea, vomiting, and diarrhea. Other symptoms include headache, stiff neck, upset stomach, confusion, or convulsions. |
| Patient Management | Care is mostly supportive, concentrating on the symptoms. Listeriosis may be treated with antibiotics. |
| Protective Measures | Since listeriosis is transmitted via contaminated food, risk of person-to-person transmission during patient care would not be expected. BSI and hand washing are indicated as with any patient. |
| Immunizations | There is currently no vaccine for listeriosis. |
| Incubation Period | Time from exposure to major symptoms can vary from a few days to approximately three weeks though gastrointestinal symptoms may begin much sooner. |
| Health Care Providers | Listeriosis is not considered a great threat to health care providers. |

# *L*YME DISEASE

| | |
|---|---|
| Causative Agent | Lyme disease is caused by *Borrelia burgdorferi.* |
| Body Systems Affected | The skin, musculoskeletal system (especially the joints), central nervous system, and cardiovascular system may be affected by lyme disease. |
| Susceptibility | Susceptibility for lyme disease is general though those persons in areas of high tick infestations have more opportunity for exposure. |
| Routes of Transmission | Lyme disease is a tickborne disease. Major reservoirs are mice and deer. |
| Signs and Symptoms | Symptoms of lyme disease occur in phases. First, a painless skin lesion at the site of the bite appears followed quickly by flu-like symptoms with weakness, stiff neck, and myalgia. Later, multiple skin lesions appear and nervous system symptoms (including meningitis, peripheral neuropathy, and Bell's palsy) commence. Cardiovascular symptoms including myocarditis, left ventricular block, and atrioventricular block are possible, though the latter is more common. In later stages, patients can develop chronic arthritis, depression, and sleep disorders. |
| Patient Management | Patient management is supportive. Antibiotic therapy may be indicated. |
| Protective Measures | There is no evidence of person-to-person transmission of lyme disease. However, health care providers should be alert to the presence of ticks which may be on the patient's clothing or body. |

**Immunizations**

A vaccine was first made available in December, 1998. The CDC recommends that the decision to vaccinate be based on geographic risk and individual exposure to tick-infested habitats. Since the vaccine is not 100% effective, health care providers who opt to take the vaccine should continue to protect themselves against contact with ticks and take appropriate precautions.

**Incubation Period**

Incubation period for lyme disease varies between 3–32 days.

**Health Care Providers**

Out-of-hospital health care providers, especially those who work in wilderness areas, should be aware of the presence of ticks.

# MEASLES (RUBEOLA, HARD MEASLES)

**Causative Agent**

Measles is caused by the measles virus, of the genus *Morbilli*.

**Body Systems Affected**

Measles affects the respiratory, integumentary, and central nervous systems, as well as the eyes.

**Susceptibility**

Though measles is considered a childhood disease, susceptibility is general.

**Routes of Transmission**

Measles may be spread by direct contact with nasal or throat secretions of infected persons. It can also be transmitted by airborne transmission.

**Signs and Symptoms**

Symptoms of measles typically appear in two stages. During the first stage, the patient may have a slight fever, runny nose, conjuctivitis, **photophobia**, malaise, and cough. A day or two before the generalized rash so commonly associated with measles appears, the patient may develop **Koplik's spots** inside the mouth. The generalized rash is red, slightly bumpy, and spreads from the head and face to the lower extremities within about three days and disappears within about six days. Some patients develop pneumonia, eye damage, and myocarditis.

**Patient Management**

There is no specific treatment for measles. Care is aimed at minimizing symptoms.

**Protective Measures**

Health care providers should observe body substance isolation and good hand washing techniques.

**Immunizations**

An immunization against measles is available.

**Incubation Period**

Symptoms usually appear within 10–12 days of exposure although a range of 8–13 days is possible.

**Health Care Providers**

Since measles is one of the most highly contagious infectious diseases, health care providers should assure immunity. In general, one may be considered immune if he/she meets one or more of the following criteria:

- has received at least one dose of live measles vaccine after first birthday
- has documentation of prior physician-diagnosed measles
- has had laboratory testing which indicates immunity
- was born before 1957

# MENINGOCOCCAL MENINGITIS

**Causative Agent**

Meningitis may be bacterial, viral, or fungal. Meningococcal (spinal) meningitis is caused by *Neisseria meningitidis* bacteria.

**Body Systems Affected**

Meningitis affects the respiratory and central nervous systems.

**Susceptibility**

Susceptibility to meningitis is general, thought it has been suggested that children under 5 years, teenagers and young adults, and older people are at greater risk.

**Routes of Transmission**

Transmission is by direct contact with a patient's respiratory secretions or through airborne transmission of respiratory droplets. The bacteria does not survive very long outside the body.

**Signs and Symptoms**

Onset is rapid. Symptoms include headache, fever, chills, vomiting, neck stiffness, joint pain, **nuchal rigidity**, and **petechial rash**. Some patients develop septic shock.

**Patient Management**

Care is primarily supportive. Pharmacologic therapy with rifampin, spiramycin, minocycline, ceftriaxone, or ciprofloxacin may be indicated.

**Protective Measures**

Body substance isolation is indicated, including masking both the caregiver and patient if feasible. Effective hand washing is important.

**Immunizations**

Vaccines are available which are effective against several strains of meningitis.

**Incubation Period**

Patients can carry the bacteria for days, weeks, or months before symptoms appear.

| Health Care Providers | Health care providers should be alert to the possibility of direct transmission though contaminated linen and airway equipment. Both BSI and respiratory protection are necessary. |
| --- | --- |

# ℳONONUCLEOSIS

| Causative Agent | Mononucleosis is a viral disease caused by the Epstein-Barr virus. It affects certain types of white blood cells. |
| --- | --- |
| Body Systems Affected | Mononucleosis affects the oropharnyx, tonsils, and respiratory system. |
| Susceptibility | Susceptibility is general. Prior infection by Epstein-Barr virus generally confers a high degree of resistance. |
| Routes of Transmission | Transmission of mononucleosis is person-to-person via saliva. In rare instances, mononucleosis has been transmitted by blood transfusion. |
| Signs and Symptoms | Symptoms of mononucleosis include sore throat, fever, swollen glands, and fatigue. Sometimes the liver and spleen are affected. |
| Patient Management | Treatment for mononucleosis is primarily supportive with an emphasis on rest and drinking plenty of fluids. **Nonsteroidal anti-inflammatory drugs (NSAIDS)** may be of value in relief of symptoms. |
| Protective Measures | Health care providers should utilize good handwashing techniques and BSI. |
| Immunizations | There is no vaccine for mononucleosis. |
| Incubation Period | Symptoms of mononucleosis typically appear four to six weeks after exposure. |

**Health Care Providers**    Since the virus may be active in the patient's throat for as long as one year after infection, health care providers should be alert to the possibility of infection through direct contact with infected saliva. For this reason, health care providers should utilize BSI and observe good hand washing techniques.

# MUMPS

**Causative Agent**    Mumps is a very contagious viral disease caused by the mumps virus, of the genus *Paramyxovirus*.

**Body Systems Affected**    Mumps affects the salivary glands and may affect the central nervous system.

**Susceptibility**    Susceptibility is general. Before the mumps vaccine became widely available, nearly every child caught mumps. Though the vaccine is widely available today, those who do not take it are at risk of contracting the disease.

**Routes of Transmission**    Mumps is spread person-to-person through direct contact with infected saliva and through droplets from a cough or sneeze.

**Signs and Symptoms**    Approximately one third of patients with mumps experience no symptoms. Those with symptoms complain of severe swelling and soreness of the salivary glands in cheeks and jaw, neck or ear pain, headache, tiredness, and fever.

**Patient Management**    Care of patients with mumps is supportive. Emphasis should be placed on pushing oral fluids and bed rest. NSAIDs may be taken to control fever. Warm moist towels may be placed to relieve swelling and pain.

**Protective Measures**   BSI and effective hand washing are essential. When appropriate, the patient should be masked to reduce the chance of transmission.

**Immunizations**   A mumps vaccine is readily available and should be taken by adults born after 1956 who have no proof of immunity, health care providers, and susceptible adolescents and adults who travel abroad.

**Incubation Period**   Symptoms usually appear between 12–25 days after exposure.

**Health Care Providers**   Since infected health care providers may spread the virus to patients, they should make sure they are immune to the disease and should take care to decontaminate infected equipment and supplies after use on a patient with mumps.

# PERTUSSIS (WHOOPING COUGH)

**Causative Agent**   Pertussis is a highly contagious bacterial infection caused by the *Bordetella pertussis*.

**Body Systems Affected**   Pertussis affects the oropharynx and respiratory tract.

**Susceptibility**   Anyone exposed to the disease can be infected by pertussis. Previous infection generally confers immunity, though subsequent attacks in adolescents and adults suggests that immunity may decrease over time.

**Routes of Transmission**

Pertussis is spread by direct contact with respiratory discharges or through exposure to airborne droplets from a cough.

**Signs and Symptoms**

Initially, symptoms mimic that of the common cold and include sneezing, runny nose, cough, and mild fever. This is called the catarrhal stage. Within two weeks, the cough becomes severe and is characterized by episodes of repeated rapid coughs followed by a crowing or high-pitched whoop. It is during this paroxysmal stage that pertussis is typically diagnosed. The whoop may not be present in infants under six months and adults. Thick clear mucous may be discharged. Symptoms may continue for one to two months and will typically be milder in older adults. Recovery is gradual. During the last, or convalescent, stage the cough becomes less paroxysmal and disappears over 2–3 weeks.

**Patient Management**

Care is primarily supportive. Antibiotics, including erythromycin, may be helpful in decreasing the period of communicability.

**Protective Measures**

Caregivers should utilize body substance isolation and thorough hand washing techniques. Care should be taken when handling linens contaminated with respiratory secretions.

**Immunizations**

A vaccination against pertussis is included in the DTP and DtaP vaccines. Prior infection with pertussis typically confers prolonged immunity.

**Incubation Period**

The typical incubation period is 5–10 days though it may be as long as 21 days.

**Health Care Providers**   Since many cases of pertussis are misdiagnosed as colds or flu, the health care provider should consistently utilize BSI and good hand washing procedures. Care should be taken in handling infected linens and respiratory equipment and supplies.

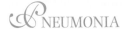 **NEUMONIA**

**Causative Agent**   Over three million cases of pneumonia are reported each year in the United States. Up to one-third of these cases are hospitalized, which accounts for 10% of adult acute care hospital admissions in the United States. Pneumonia may be bacterial, viral, or fungal. Viral pneumonia is rare in adults except during outbreaks. Bacterial sources of pneumonia include *Streptococcus pneumoniae, Mycoplasma pneumoniae, Staphylococcus aureus, H. influenzae, Klebsiella pneumoniae, Moraxella catarrhalis,* and *Legionella* (Figure 5-5).

---

- *Streptococcus pneumoniae*
- *Mycoplasma pneumoniae*
- *Staphylococcus aureus*
- *H. influenzae*
- *Klebsiella pneumoniae*
- *Moraxella catarrhalis*
- *Legionella*

---

FIGURE 5-5 Bacterial sources of pneumonia. Pneumonia may be caused by one of many possible sources.

**Body Systems Affected**   Pneumonia affects the respiratory and central nervous system. It may also affect the ears, nose, and throat.

**Susceptibility**   Anyone exposed to the disease can catch pneumonia, though certain groups may be considered more susceptible due to decreased resistance to the disease. These groups include those who are elderly, have significant pre-existing illness, or those who are immunocompromised.

**Routes of Transmission**   Pneumonia is spread through respiratory exposure to droplets from a sneeze or cough, or direct contact to objects contaminated with respiratory secretions of those who have pneumonia.

**Signs and Symptoms**   Persons who have pneumonia complain of sudden onset of chills, fever, chest discomfort, and shortness of breath. Coughs may be productive with yellow-green phlegm. In children, be alert to high fever, tachycardia, and chest retractions, which are ominous signs.

**Patient Management**   Initial care is primarily supportive. Antibiotics, including erythromycin, doxycycline, augmentin, cephalosporin, or vacomycin may be used.

**Protective Measures**   As with any patient, PPE should be used and hand washing after patient contact should be thorough.

**Immunizations**   A vaccine that protects against some causes of pneumonia is currently available. Though it will not protect against pneumonia of every cause, it will protect against approximately 88% of pneumococcal bacteria that cause pneumonia. Immunity is better for younger people and the immunity lasts up to 10 years for most people.

**Incubation Period**

Most experts agree that the incubation period for pneumonia may be as short as 1–3 days.

**Health Care Providers**

Since health care providers are often called upon to treat patients with pneumococcal disease, they should consider taking the vaccine. BSI is essential, as is careful hand washing. Linens and other materials contaminated with respiratory secretions should be treated as infectious and disinfected accordingly.

# ABIES

**Causative Agent**

Rabies is a viral disease of the central nervous system. The causative agent, rabies virus of the genus *Lyssavirus*, is found in domestic and wild animals.

**Body Systems Affected**

Rabies affects the central nervous system.

**Susceptibility**

Susceptibility is general for anyone who is bitten by an infected animal.

**Routes of Transmission**

Humans most frequently become infected with rabies through the virus-laden saliva from the scratch or bite of an infected animal. Person-to-person transmission is theoretically possible though no case has been documented.

**Signs and Symptoms**

Symptoms of rabies typically present in three phases. During the **prodromal** phase, the patient presents with fever, pharyngitis, headache, anorexia, and pain, or **paresthesia**, at the site of the bite or scratch. These symptoms usually last two to ten days. The second, or neurologic stage, presents with aphasia, paresis, paralysis, lack of coordination, mental status changes, and hyperactivity. Third stage symptoms may include hypotension, coma, cardiac arrhythmias, disseminated intravascular coagulation (DIC), cardiac arrest, and death.

Other nonspecific signs of rabies include myoclonus, hypersalivation, agitation, anxiety, and increased lacrimation.

**Patient Management**

Management of rabies includes thorough debridement of the wound, drainage as necessary, and vigorous cleaning of the wound with soap and water followed by irrigation with 70% alcohol. Human rabies immune globin (HRIG) should be administered and patients should be immunized with human diploid cell vaccine (HDCV) or rabies vaccine. Tetanus prophylaxis and antibiotics should be administered as indicated.

**Protective Measures**

Though transmission from human patients to health care providers has never been documented, BSI should be utilized and thorough hand washing should take place.

**Immunizations**

Rabies vaccine is available as a human diploid-cell vaccine (HDCV) and an adsorbed vaccine (RVA). Immunization is typically directed toward individuals with high probability of exposure.

**Incubation Period**

The incubation period of rabies is usually between 3–8 weeks although it may be as few as five days or as long as one year, or longer.

**Health Care Providers**   Though human-to-human transmission has not been documented, BSI should be utilized and handwashing should be thorough. EMS workers and those who work in wilderness or other outdoor settings should be especially cautious when dealing with and working around animals. The animal source of reported rabies cases is most commonly raccoons, bats, skunks, foxes, and dogs.

# ℛocky Mountain Spotted Fever

**Causative Agent**   Rocky Mountain Spotted Fever (RMSF) is caused by a specialized bacteria called *Rickettsia rickettsii*.

**Body Systems Affected**   Major complications associated with RMSF include kidney failure and shock. The liver and lungs may also be affected.

**Susceptibility**   Susceptibility is general, but those who work outdoors and have greater opportunity for exposure to ticks are more likely to be infected. RMSF has been reported throughout the United States with the exception of Alaska, Hawaii, and Maine. Most cases are reported in the eastern U.S.

**Routes of Transmission**   Transmission is typically from the bite of an infected tick or by contamination of broken skin with the body fluids of a tick crushed while still attached. Person-to-person transmission is possible through transfusion of infected blood, although transmission through this route is extremely rare.

| | |
|---|---|
| **Signs and Symptoms** | Patients frequently complain of fever, headache, tiredness, nausea and vomiting, and deep muscle pain. The rash associated with RMSF may begin on the legs or arms, and may rapidly spread to the rest of the body. The rash initially appears as small red spots or blotches and may later change to look more like bruises or bloody patches under the skin. |
| **Patient Management** | Initial treatment is supportive. Antibiotic therapy with tetracycline or chloramphenicol may be effective. |
| **Protective Measures** | Though RMSF is not contagious person-to-person, BSI and effective hand washing is indicated as with any patient. |
| **Immunizations** | There is no vaccine for RMSF at this time. |
| **Incubation Period** | Symptoms of RMSF typically begin 3–12 days after a tick bite though they may occur as early as one day or as many as 14 days after exposure. |
| **Health Care Providers** | Though the risk of person-to-person transmission is very minor, health care providers who work in outdoor and wilderness areas should be alert to the possibility of ticks and should check themselves for ticks frequently, utilize insect repellants, and dress appropriate to the environment for maximal tick protection. |

# RUBELLA (GERMAN MEASLES)

| | |
|---|---|
| **Causative Agent** | Rubella is an infectious disease caused by the rubella virus. |
| **Body Systems Affected** | Rubella affects the respiratory, integumentary, musculoskeletal, and lymphatic systems. |

**Susceptibility**

After the loss of maternal antibodies, susceptibility for rubella is general. Maternal transmission to the fetus is the greatest risk because the rubella virus can cause developmental defects. Natural infection and immunization generally confer life-long immunity.

**Routes of Transmission**

Rubella virus is passed from person to person by direct contact with nasopharyngeal secretions or by inhalation of droplets from a sneeze or cough. Infants with **congenital rubella syndrome (CRS)** shed large amounts of the virus in their secretions so these secretions are highly contagious.

**Signs and Symptoms**

Typical symptoms include a rash on the face and neck that spreads to the limbs and trunk (Figure 5-6). This rash is not easily seen on dark-skinned individuals. Infected persons also may experience a slight fever with a runny nose and sore throat, enlarged lymph nodes, and red eyes. Children typically have no serious side effects, though rubella in adults is considerably more serious. Younger females sometimes develop a self-limiting arthritis. More extreme side effects include **encephalitis, thrombocytopaenia**, and **Gullain-Barre syndrome.** The most serious hazard is to the unborn child who may suffer from heart defects, hearing impairment, and cataracts. Multiple defects are fairly common and spontaneous abortion is possible.

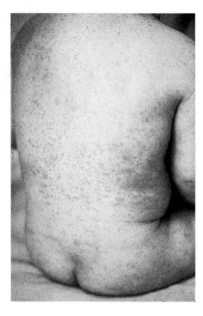

**FIGURE 5-6** Rubella rash. (Photo courtesy of the Centers for Disease Control and Prevention.)

**Patient Management**

Rubella is typically self-correcting so treatment is rarely necessary. Care is primarily supportive, and is concentrated on controlling any fever and keeping the patient comfortable. When complications exist, they may need more aggressive treatment.

**Protective Measures**

When caring for a patient with rubella, BSI is indicated and effective hand washing is recommended.

**Immunizations**

The vaccine available for rubella is 98–99% effective and is combined with the mumps and measles vaccines (MMR). It is not recommended for pregnant females and it is suggested that females who take the vaccine not become pregnant within one month after vaccination. The vaccine is not recommended for persons with a weakened immune system.

**Incubation Period**

Incubation period for rubella is 12–23 days though symptoms typically appear within 16–18 days.

**Health Care Providers**

Health care providers should be screened for immunity and immunized as necessary. Females of child-bearing age should be immunized due to the risk of infecting an unborn baby. BSI should be observed and effective hand washing should take place.

# SALMONELLOSIS

**Causative Agent**

*Salmonella* is a bacteria that infects the gastrointestinal tract and the blood. Salmonellosis is a bacterial infection caused by one of the more than 2,000 strands of *Salmonella*.

**Body Systems Affected**

Salmonellosis affects the gastrointestinal system and blood.

**Susceptibility**

Susceptibility for salmonellosis is general though children, the elderly, and those with a depressed immune system are at greater risk.

**Routes of Transmission**

Salmonellosis is typically considered a foodborne disease acquired through eating contaminated eggs, unpasteurized dairy products, or raw poultry. It may also be transmitted though contact with infected animals, especially turtles, iguanas, and other reptiles.

| | |
|---|---|
| **Signs and Symptoms** | People who have salmonellosis complain of fever, chills, diarrhea, abdominal discomfort, and vomiting. |
| **Patient Management** | Care for salmonellosis is largely supportive. Fluids may be required to prevent dehydration. |
| **Protective Measures** | As with any patient, BSI should be utilized. Effective hand washing is essential. |
| **Immunizations** | There is no available vaccine for salmonellosis at this time. |
| **Incubation Period** | The expected incubation period for salmonellosis is 1–3 days. |
| **Health Care Providers** | Health care providers should be alert to the possibility of the disease, and should take BSI precautions and practice good hand washing with all patients. Since reptiles, particularly iguanas have become popular pets, health care providers should be alert to the possibility of *Salmonella* infection. |

# CABIES

| | |
|---|---|
| **Causative Agent** | The causative agent of scabies is *Sarcoptes scabiei*, a small **mite** that burrows into the skin. Scabies are grayish in color, nearly transparent and about the size of the period at the end of this sentence. |
| **Body Systems Affected** | Scabies affect the integumentary system. The mites typically begin by burrowing into the webs between fingers and toes, around the wrist, or navel. Later, the mites spread to other areas including the groin, armpits, abdomen, and elbows. |

| | |
|---|---|
| **Susceptibility** | Susceptibility is general. Scabies does not discriminate in regard to age, race, or socioeconomic standing. Those who have been previously exposed may develop fewer mites and tend to develop symptoms faster (in 1–4 days versus 2–6 weeks for those who have never been exposed). |
| **Routes of Transmission** | Scabies is most frequently spread by direct skin-to-skin contact. It is possible to catch scabies indirectly through contaminated bedclothes and undergarments, but only if these items were contaminated by an infected person immediately prior. Scabies may also be transmitted during sexual contact. It takes approximately 2–3 minutes for a mite to burrow into the skin. |
| **Signs and Symptoms** | The primary symptom of scabies is itching. People who become sensitive to the presence of scabies or their waste products may develop large areas of reddened, inflamed, itching skin. |
| **Patient Management** | Care is largely supportive and includes replacing contaminated clothing. Skin lotions containing lindane, permethrin, or crotamiton may be prescribed to control the itching. |
| **Protective Measures** | BSI is essential. All linens and contaminated clothing should be bagged. |
| **Immunizations** | There is no vaccination for scabies at this time. |
| **Incubation Period** | Symptoms appear 2–6 weeks after exposure to scabies. An infected person will continue to spread scabies until all mites and eggs are destroyed. |

**Health Care Providers**   Those who care for patients with scabies should take care to wear appropriate PPE, bag linens and contaminated clothing, and decontaminate all equipment that comes in contact with the patient.

# 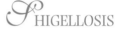HIGELLOSIS

**Causative Agent**   Shigellosis is a bacterial infection that affects the lining of the intestinal tract, caused by infection with *Shigella* organisms.

**Body Systems Affected**   Shigellosis affects the gastrointestinal system and liver.

**Susceptibility**   Susceptibility for shigellosis is general though more cases are reported in the summer months in areas with a cooler climate. The disease tends to be more common in children, ages 2–3 years.

**Routes of Transmission**   This disease is most commonly spread through direct person-to-person contact with infected stool. Water and food may become contaminated, which allows an opportunity for waterborne and foodborne transmission. When sexual practices allow contact with stool, opportunity also exists for sexual transmission.

**Signs and Symptoms**   Patients with shigellosis experience diarrhea, abdominal cramps, nausea and vomiting, painful bowel movements, fever, and loss of appetite.

**Patient Management**   Aggressive treatment for shigellosis is rarely indicated. IV fluids are sometimes needed to combat dehydration. Antibiotics may be helpful in severe cases.

**Protective Measures**       BSI and thorough hand washing are indicated.

**Immunizations**             There is currently no vaccine for shigellosis.

**Incubation Period**         The incubation period for shigellosis ranges from 1–7 days with the average being 2–3 days.

**Health Care Providers**     Health care providers should always observe BSI and take care to isolate themselves from potentially infected feces. Hand washing is, as always, very important.

# YPHILIS

**Causative Agent**           Syphilis is caused by the *Treponema pallidum* bacteria. An infection is caused first at the initially exposed site, then moves throughout the body, causing damage to multiple organs over time.

**Body Systems Affected**     Syphilis affects many organs including the skin, eyes, and kidneys as well as the cardiovascular, skeletal, and central nervous systems.

**Susceptibility**            Susceptibility to syphilis is general. Approximately 30% of exposures result in infection.

**Routes of Transmission**    This disease is transmitted from the initial ulcer of an infected person to the skin or mucous membranes of the genital area, the mouth, or the anus of the sexual partner. It can also penetrate broken skin on other parts of the body. It may also be passed from a pregnant woman to her unborn child or transmitted via needle-stick or blood transfusion.

**Signs and Symptoms**    Syphilis presents in four stages (primary, secondary, latent, and tertiary). The first symptom of primary syphilis is the development of a **chancre** ulcer. This chancre usually develops in 3–6 weeks after the initial exposure and is located on the part of the body initially exposed. If untreated, the disease may progress to the secondary stage.

Secondary syphilis is noted for its skin rash, which may occur on any part of the body but nearly always includes the palms of the hands and soles of the feet. The rash presents as small red or brown lesions that contain active bacteria. Any contact with the broken skin of an infected person may spread the infection during this stage. Other symptoms include headache, fever, sore throat, fatigue, and swollen lymph nodes. Symptoms may continue sporadically for one to two years and may progress to latent syphilis if untreated.

Latent syphilis is a stage in which the syphilis is no longer contagious and no symptoms are present. Some patients relapse into secondary syphilis while others may progress to tertiary syphilis. There are usually no more relapses after four years.

The fourth stage, tertiary syphilis, can last for years or even decades. Complications include mental illness, blindness, central nervous system problems, heart disease, and even death.

| | |
|---|---|
| **Patient Management** | Antibiotics such as penicillin, erythromycin, and doxyclycline may be helpful. Other care is supportive. |
| **Protective Measures** | Strict BSI and thorough hand washing are essential. Caution should be used when handling soiled linens. |
| **Immunizations** | There is currently no vaccine for syphilis. |
| **Incubation Period** | Symptoms of syphilis may occur in as few as 10 days or as long as three months. |
| **Health Care Providers** | Health care providers should take care to avoid exposure to any body fluid, including the fluid from lesions. BSI and effective hand washing are essential. |

# $\mathcal{T}$ETANUS

| | |
|---|---|
| **Causative Agent** | Tetanus is an infection caused by *Clostridium tetani*, a bacteria found in almost anything lying on the ground, including the soil. *C. tetani* seems to thrive on rusty metal, so puncture wounds with rusty nails are a common cause of tetanus. *C. tetani* readily grows in wounds and produces a toxin that paralyzes muscles. |
| **Body Systems Affected** | Tetanus generally affects the musculoskeletal system by causing muscular stiffness and rigidity (Figure 5-7). |
| **Susceptibility** | Susceptibility is general. |
| **Routes of Transmission** | Tetanus can not be transmitted from person to person. It is generally transmitted through puncture wounds or cuts. |

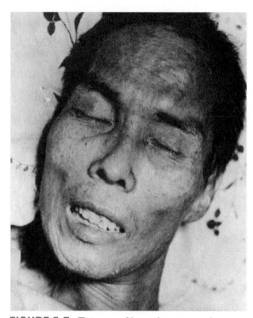

FIGURE 5-7  Tetanus. Note the muscular contraction of the jaw. (Photo courtesy of the Centers for Disease Control and Prevention.)

**Signs and Symptoms**

Symptoms of tetanus include fever, headache, difficulty in swallowing, and muscular stiffness in the neck and jaw (thus the name lockjaw).

**Patient Management**

Care for patients experiencing symptoms of tetanus is mostly supportive.

**Protective Measures**

Since tetanus is not communicable from person to person, only routine measures are necessary.

**Immunizations**

Two agents are available. Tetanus immune globulin (TIG) is a concentrate of antibodies produced against tetanus toxin by immunized people. Another available agent is tetanus toxoid, which works by making the body produce antibodies to the toxin and protect one from future infections. Since immunity to tetanus wanes with time, periodic boosters are necessary.

**Incubation Period**

The incubation period for tetanus is typically 8 days, but may range from 3 days to 3 weeks.

**Health Care Providers**

Health care providers may have opportunity to counsel patients who may have been exposed to *Clostridium tetani*. Patients who have received a small cut or puncture wound may defer treatment due to the perceived minor nature of the wound. Patients should be made aware of the danger of tetanus and of the importance of immunization.

# TUBERCULOSIS

**Causative Agent**

Tuberculosis is a bacterial disease caused by *Mycobacterium tuberculosis*.

**Body Systems Affected**

Tuberculosis can attack any part of the body. Though it usually affects the lungs, it can also affect the renal, musculoskeletal, or lymphatic systems.

**Susceptibility**

Anyone can get tuberculosis, though immunocompromised persons and elderly persons are at greater risk. Those with diabetes or cancer may also be more susceptible.

**Routes of Transmission**

Person-to-person transmission of tuberculosis is primarily through inhalation of droplets from a sneeze or cough. Persons may also become exposed to tuberculosis through prolonged, close exposure to an infected person. There are also a few recorded cases of exposure through direct infection through mucous membranes or broken skin, though this type exposure is uncommon.

**Signs and Symptoms**

Common symptoms include a persistent cough, fever, weight loss, fatigue, and night sweats. Some infected persons have no symptoms.

**Patient Management**

Initial care is primarily supportive. Recommended therapeutic care includes administration of a combination of medications that may include Isoniazid, Rifampin, Ethambutol, Pyrazinamide, and Streptomycin.

**Protective Measures**

HEPA respirators should be worn when in contact with patients who have active tuberculosis.

**Immunizations**

There is currently no vaccine for tuberculosis. A skin test (**Mantoux test**) can show if TB bacteria are present.

**Incubation Period**

The incubation period for tuberculosis is typically between 4–12 weeks.

**Health Care Providers**

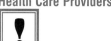

Health care providers, especially those in the prehospital or out-of-hospital setting, should be aware of the possibility of contracting TB from patients with an active cough. In situations where a caregiver will be in a confined area with the patient for a prolonged period of time, caregivers should wear HEPA mask. Unless contraindicated by medical conditions, it is also advisable to place a mask on the patient.

## CASE STUDY 5.1

Your patient is a 46-year-old male who complains of fever, bloody diarrhea, abdominal cramps, and vomiting over a two-day period. The patient works in the poultry industry and has regular contact with young fowl.

### REFLECT AND CONSIDER

➤ Based on the patient's occupation, what is the most likely source of his illness?

➤ What other illnesses are his signs and symptoms consistent with?

➤ What precautions would you take when treating this patient?

## CASE STUDY 5.2

Your patient is a 33-year-old female who presents with fever and rash. The patient's symptoms began five days ago when she began to feel nauseated. The following day she developed fever, headache, and body ache. Yesterday, a rash began on her neck. The rash spread to her head, face, arms, and trunk. In the emergency room, the patient had a temperature of 102.8°F, rash, cough, and small white punctate lesions on the buccal mucosa.

### REFLECT AND CONSIDER

➤ What is the likely diagnosis for this patient?

➤ What questions would you ask the patient about her past medical history?

*(continued)*

> ➤ How could her disease be transmitted? What precautions should you take?
> ➤ Would you have taken the same precautions had the patient presented four days ago with nausea, headache, fever, and body ache? Why or why not?

## QUESTIONS FOR DISCUSSION

1. Which infectious diseases should health care providers be most concerned with?
2. Experts have said it is 200 times easier to become infected with hepatitis B than with HIV. Why?
3. Why is it important to wear a mask when working in an area infested by rodents?
4. Explain how the three types of lice are spread.
5. Describe each of the four stages of syphilis.
6. What infectious disease is sometimes referred to as lockjaw? Why?
7. Why is hepatitis C a serious threat to health care providers?
8. Why is legionellosis sometimes referred to as Legionaire's Disease?

## WORTH THINKING ABOUT

- Does the nature of your work (e.g., frequent overseas travel, working outdoors) dictate that you take extra precautions against any particular diseases?

## BIBLIOGRAPHY

Centers for Disease Control and Prevention. (1989, June 23). Guidelines for prevention of transmission of human immunodeficiency virus and hepatis B virus to health-care and public safety workers. *Morbidity and Mortality Weekly Report 38* (S-6).

Centers for Disease Control and Prevention. (1999, Dec. 31). Summary of notifiable diseases, United States, 1998. *Morbidity and Mortality Weekly Report 47*(53).

Centers for Disease Control and Prevention. (2000, Feb. 4). Outbreaks of salmonella serotype enteritidis infection associated with eating raw or undercooked shell eggs–United States, 1996-1998. *Morbidity and Mortality Weekly Report 49* (4).

Centers for Disease Control and Prevention. (2000, March 17). Hantavirus pulmonary syndrome—Panama, 1999-2000. *Morbidity and Mortality Weekly Report 49* (10).

Centers for Disease Control and Prevention. (2000, April 14). Salmonellosis associated with chicks and ducklings—Michigan and Missouri, Spring, 1999. *Morbidity and Mortality Weekly Report 49* (14).

Centers for Disease Control and Prevention. (2000, April 21). *Escherichia coli* 0111:H8 outbreak among teenage campers—Texas, 1999. *Morbidity and Mortality Weekly Report 49* (15).

Centers for Disease Control and Prevention. Web site. http://www.cdc.gov.

Cockrum, E. L. (1997). *Rabies, lyme disease, Hantavirus and other animal-borne human diseases in the United States and Canada.* Tucson, AZ: Fisher Books.

Damjanov, I. (2000). *Pathology for the health-related professions.* Philadelphia, PA: W.B. Saunders.

Epimmune. Web site. http://www.epimmune.com.

The Hepatitis Information Network. Web site. http://www.hepnet.com.

Kids Health. Web site. http://www.kidshealth.org.

National Fire Academy, (1992). *Infection control for emergency response personnel: The supervisor's role.* Emmitsburg, MD: Author.

Neighbors, M., & Tannehill-Jones, R. (2000). *Human diseases*. Albany, NY: Delmar.

New York State Department of Health. Web site. http://www.health.state.ny.us.

NZ Dermnet. Web site. http://www.dermnet.org.nz.

Smith, P. W. (1994). *Infection control in long-term care facilities*. (2nd ed.). Albany, NY: Delmar.

South Dakota Department of Health. Web site. http://www.state.sd.us/doh.

Sugar, A. M., & Lyman, C. A. (1997). *A practical guide to medically important fungi and the diseases they cause*. Philadelphia, PA: Lippincott-Raven.

Thibodeau, G. A., & Patton, K. T. (1999). *Anatomy and physiology*. (4th ed.). St. Louis, MO: Mosby.

Web MD Health. Web site. http://www.webmd.com.

World Health Organization. Web site. http://www.who.int.

# Chapter 6
# Protection from Communicable Disease

▼ ▼ ▼ ▼ ▼ ▼ ▼

## LEARNING OBJECTIVES

After completing this chapter, the reader should be able to:

- list and describe common engineering controls and work practices.
- discuss the importance of personal health to the health care provider.
- discuss the risks, benefits, and side effects of the hepatitis B vaccine.
- list the vaccines recommended for health care providers by the CDC.
- discuss the proper disposal of contaminated supplies.
- demonstrate the disinfection of patient care areas.
- demonstrate the disinfection of patient care equipment.
- demonstrate proper use of personal protective equipment.
- demonstrate proper hand washing technique.

## KEY TERMS

- airborne precautions
- biohazard container
- body substance isolation (BSI)
- contact precautions
- droplet precautions
- engineering controls
- essential functions
- HEPA (high efficiency particulate air) respirator
- nosocomial infections
- personal health
- personal protective equipment
- pre-entry physical exam
- safe work practices
- sharps containers
- standard precautions
- transmission-based precautions

## INTRODUCTION

Protection from communicable disease is a joint responsibility of the employer and the employee. This chapter addresses the responsibilities of each and how the employer and employee must work together to achieve optimal protection.

## ENGINEERING CONTROLS

**Engineering controls** are actions taken by the employer to make the workplace safer by engineering safety directly into the workplace. This may include anything from placement of sharps containers and hand washing facilities to providing adequate storage facilities for hazardous chemicals. This may entail making the surfaces of work areas easy to clean and sanitize, or installing adequate air handling and ventilation equipment. In short, engineering controls make safe practices practical and convenient for the employee.

## Hand Washing Facilities

Hand washing facilities, including hot water, soap, and a mechanism for drying should be made available and accessible to all health care providers. When traditional hand washing is impractical, waterless hand washing solutions and paper towels should be made available.

## Biohazard Containers

The employer must also provide readily accessible **biohazard containers** (Figure 6-1) for the disposal of contaminated materials. Sometimes called **sharps containers**, these closable, puncture resistant containers are used to dispose of contaminated needles, scalpels, and sutures. OSHA's bloodborne pathogen standard requires these containers to not only be closable and puncture resistant, but to also be leakproof on the sides and bottom, and to be labeled or color coded in accordance with the standard.

OSHA also requires that sharps containers be:

- easily accessible and located near the area where sharps are used.

- maintained upright throughout use.

- replaced routinely and not be allowed to become overfilled.

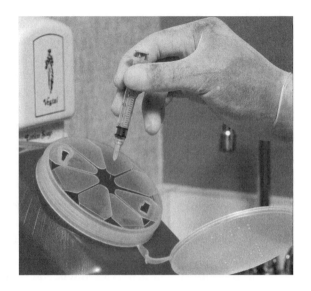

FIGURE 6-1  Biohazard container used for proper disposal of sharp objects such as IV needles.

When sharps containers are moved, OSHA requires that they be closed (to prevent spillage) and, if leakage is possible, placed in a secondary container that must be closable and constructed in such a way as to contain its contents and prevent leakage during handling or transport.

## Medical Devices

In recent years medical device manufacturers have worked toward engineering safety directly into such devices as needles, syringes, and diagnostic equipment (Figure 6-2). Intravenous placement sets are now available, which offer extra protection by allowing the needle to be retracted into a secure container before being detached from the patient catheter. Some blood-drawing needles have the feature of shielding the needle before it is withdrawn from the vein or artery.

Syringes are being made with protective shields to cover the needle or with needles that retract into the barrel of the syringe after use.

According to the National Institute for Occupational Safety and Health (NIOSH), protected-needle and needleless IV systems have decreased needlestick injuries caused by attaching a syringe to an IV connector by as much as 88%. Studies also show that phlebotomy (blood-drawing) injuries were reduced by 82% through the use of a needle shield.

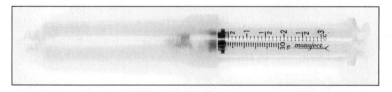

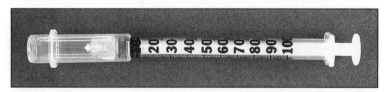

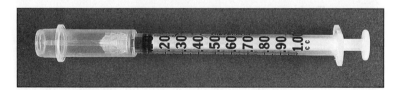

**FIGURE 6-2** Medical devices with built-in safety features.

Health care providers should remember that improved medical devices are engineered with safety in mind but are not a replacement for safe work practices or individuals taking care with their work.

## Other Concerns

Eye wash stations, when applicable, should be accessible and maintained in good working condition. Care should be taken to assure that eye wash stations are placed in appropriate locations and that all employees understand how to operate them.

When potentially hazardous chemicals (including many cleaning compounds) are used, they must be properly labeled and stored in appropriate locations near where they are used. Material Safety Data Sheets (MSDS), which give persons working with or responding to emergencies involving chemicals specific information on physical properties, toxicity, and first aid, must be available and accessible to those who use the chemicals in their work.

Engineering controls are considered the responsibility of the employer, but the employee is responsible to notify the employer of engineering controls that are necessary to promote safe work practices.

## SAFE WORK PRACTICES

**Safe work practices** are typically considered a responsibility of the employee. The employer however, is responsible to assure compliance with these practices. Safe work practices should be listed in the employer's standard operating procedure or employee handbook. Figure 6-3 shows examples of common safe work practices.

- The employee must not eat or drink while in a work area.
- The employee must not smoke while in a work area.
- The employee must not handle contact lenses in a work area.
- The employee must not apply makeup or lip balm in a work area.
- The employee must wash hands after contact with each patient.
- The employee must wear appropriate protective equipment when providing patient care.

FIGURE 6-3  Examples of safe work practices.

## Hand Washing

Hand washing is arguably the most important work practice and is cited by the Association for Professionals in Infection Control and Epidemiology as being the single most important work practice for preventing nosocomial infections. Figure 6-4 features a listing of hand washing tips.

- Wash your hands. It is the single most important procedure for preventing nosocomial infections.
- Wash your hands after prolonged or intense contact with any patient.
- Wash your hands before and after situations where contamination is likely.
- Wash your hands after removing gloves.
- When in doubt, wash your hands.

FIGURE 6-4  Hand washing tips. (Source: Association for Professionals in Infection Control and Epidemiology, Inc.)

Employees should be instructed in proper hand washing techniques and employers should assure compliance with proper hand washing procedures. Employees should wash their hands for at least 15 seconds with soap and running warm water before and after each contact with a patient and after removing gloves. One of the greatest problems with hand washing is that when improperly done, the employee's hands can be contaminated before the hand washing procedure is complete. Figure 6-5 outlines a suggested hand washing technique that will help prevent recontamination.

OSHA recognizes that some work areas, especially outside the hospital, may not have access to running water. In these cases, the employer must provide antiseptic towelettes or hand cleaner and a clean cloth or paper towels to accommodate hand washing. Though these products work very well, the health care provider should wash hands with soap and running water as soon after use as is practical.

## Handling and Using Sharps

Needles, sutures, and scalpels are common tools of the trade for many health care providers. Due to the possibility of injury and contamination through accidental cuts and sticks with these devices, health care providers should use extreme care when working with or disposing of these items. Over 800,000 needlestick incidents occur each year in U.S. hospitals. Many of these incidents occur after the needle was used and approximately 1/3 occur during disposal.

As a general rule, needles should be disposed of immediately after use and should not be bent or recapped. If it is necessary to recap a needle, a one-handed tech-

## Proper Hand Washing Technique

To avoid recontamination during hand washing, follow this procedure.

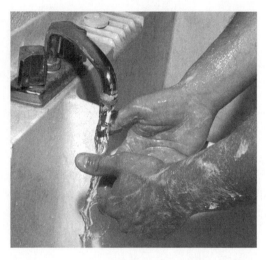

1. Make paper towel readily available. A common mistake is to wash hands and then access paper towels. This contaminates clean hands.

2. Turn water on.

3. Dispense soap. The use of liquid soap is preferred over bar soap.

4. Rub soaped hands vigorously under running water. Rinse from proximal to distal. (forearms to fingertips)

5. With the water still running, dry hands with previously dispensed towel. Use the towel to turn the water off. This will prevent you from contaminating your clean hands by touching the towel dispenser or the faucet handle.

6. Dispose of the towel in an appropriate container.

FIGURE 6-5 Suggested hand washing procedure.

nique should be used. Figure 6-6 illustrates a one-handed technique for recapping needles.

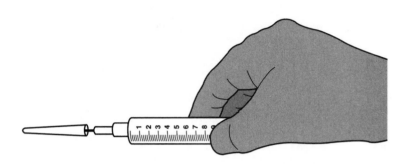

**FIGURE 6-6** One-handed technique to recap a needle. Though recapping is not recommended, use the one-handed technique when recapping is necessary.

# IN-HOSPITAL ISOLATION

As early as 1877, health care providers used the principle of isolation to combat the spread of **nosocomial infections**. Then, patients with infectious diseases were isolated from non-infected patients in an effort to control the spread of infection within the hospital population. Today, hospitals utilize a two-tiered system developed by the Centers for Disease Control and Prevention (CDC) with the same goal, but with more clearly-defined guidelines.

## Standard and Transmission-Based Precautions

The first tier, **standard precautions**, is utilized with all patients and advocates isolation from blood, non-intact skin, mucous membranes, and all body fluids with the exception of perspiration (Figure 6-7). **Transmission-**

based precautions, the second tier, are utilized with those patients known or suspected to be infected with highly transmissible or epidemiologically important pathogens. One or more of three types of transmission-based precautions may be used, depending on the way a given disease is transmitted.

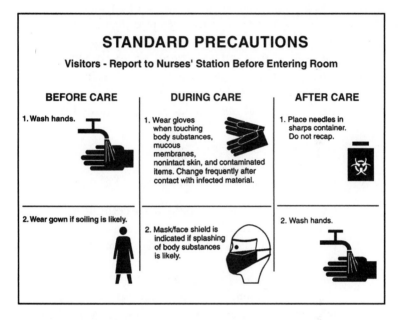

FIGURE 6-7  Standard precautions. (Courtesy of Briggs Corporation.)

Airborne Precautions

Airborne precautions are used for patients known or suspected to be infected with airborne transmissible diseases like tuberculosis and pertussis. Emphasis is placed on patient placement and respiratory protection. Patients should be isolated from other patients and placed in an area with good ventilation. Respiratory protection should be worn by all caregivers. When practical, a surgical mask should be placed on the patient during transport and times when the caregiver is in close proximity to the patient.

## Droplet Precautions

**Droplet precautions** are used to protect the health care provider from inhaling large particle droplets of moisture that carry contaminants. The patient should be isolated from other patients when possible. Health care providers should wear a mask when working within three feet of the patient. The patient should also wear a surgical mask when in close contact with the caregiver.

## Contact Precautions

**Contact precautions** deal with coming in contact with an infected person or their personal items, such as bed linens or clothing. The patient should be isolated from other patients to the extent possible. Gloves should be worn when caring for the patient and removed immediately after patient contact. Hand washing with soap and warm running water should take place after removing gloves. When it is anticipated that the caregiver will have substantial contact with the patient or his/her belongings, or when the patient is incontinent, has diarrhea, an ileostomy, a colonostomy, or drainage from a wound not controlled by a dressing, a gown should be worn. The gown should be removed and disposed of after each patient contact. Limit exposure to other patients to a minimum and use care in assuring that patient care equipment used with a patient on contact isolation is limited to use with only that patient.

# ⊘UT-OF-HOSPITAL ISOLATION

**Body substance isolation (BSI)** contends that all body substances are infectious and the employee must protect him/herself from contact with any body substance. This system of protection is generally preferred by prehospital care providers, industrial responders, and employees in many emergency departments. Emphasis is on maximal, rather than minimal, protection.

# ⊘ERSONAL PROTECTIVE EQUIPMENT

**Personal protective equipment (PPE)** is provided by the employer for use by the employee for protection from exposure to contaminants in the workplace. Personal protective equipment must be readily available at the work site or issued to employees for use.

**ALERT**

Gloves should be replaced after each patient contact.

## Gloves

Gloves are the most frequently used PPE. OSHA requires that employers provide each employee with gloves that fit properly. Persons with an allergy to latex must be provided with glove liners or non-allergenic, non-latex gloves at no cost to the employee. Gloves should be discarded and replaced as soon as practical after becoming soiled. Remember, the use of gloves does not eliminate the need to wash hands properly. The employee should wash hands immediately after removing gloves.

**ALERT**

People who wash their hands frequently and/or wear gloves often may need to use lotion to keep their hands from cracking, thereby creating a potential portal of entry for pathogens.

## Masks and Respirators

Masks should be worn when an employee may come in contact with a patient with a known airborne communicable disease and in cases where any patient is sneezing or coughing. They also may be used as an adjunct to eye protection when there is a possibility of splashing blood or body fluids.

The different types of masks available offer a vast array of protection, from the standard surgical-type mask, which provides limited protection, to HEPA respirators, which filter particles as small as 0.3 micrometers in diameter and are recommended for use when caring for tuberculosis patients (Figure 6-8). While a HEPA mask is not required on all patients, the employee should select a mask that will provide optimal protection for a given situation.

**ALERT**

HEPA (high-efficiency particulate air) respirators must be fitted to each individual's face and may not seal properly over facial hair.

## Eye Protection

Eye protection may be in the form of goggles, glasses with solid side shields, or full face shields. The employee should select the device appropriate to the situation.

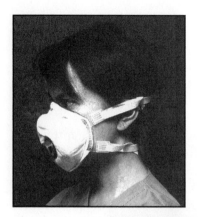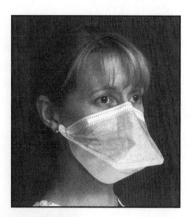

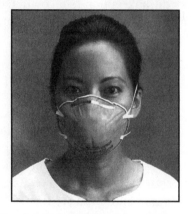

FIGURE 6-8 Masks should be selected to provide optimal protection for the situation.

Many employers require employees to wear eye protection as a precaution when caring for every patient. For this reason, some health care providers have side shields fitted to normal prescription glasses. While this may meet the requirements set forth by the employer, one should consider the additional protection that safety glasses or goggles may afford in a splash situation.

## Gowns and Protective Apparel

Gowns or additional appropriate cover should be worn in conjunction with other PPE when splash is anticipated. A uniform should not be considered PPE. Appropriate cover must be used to protect the uniform.

Many hospitals use paper or plastic gowns for this purpose. Due to the nature of the environment, these gowns may not be appropriate for use in the prehospital or industrial setting. Some pre-hospital care providers use fluid resistant paper coveralls or jackets as a more durable option to a gown. Employers should select and purchase protective equipment with the work environment in mind.

## Uniforms

If a uniform becomes soiled with blood or body fluids, the employer is responsible for its proper cleaning or replacement (at the employer's option). Due to the possibility of cross-contamination of other clothing, the employee should not launder a contaminated uniform at home. Proper laundering requires the use of a front-loading industrial washing machine connected to an approved drainage system.

Commercial laundry facilities may also be used since they typically use a combination of high water temperatures (>160°F) and chlorine bleach (50–150 parts per million) to assure the removal of harmful microorganisms. Soiled uniforms should be handled as little as possible and placed in a biohazard bag for transportation to the laundry facility.

If a pull-over shirt is contaminated it may have to be cut off to avoid unnecessary contact when pulling it over the head. If this is the case, the shirt should be cut off and placed in a biohazard bag for proper disposal. The employee should shower as soon as is practical afterwards.

# CLEAN UP

When spilled, blood and/or other body fluid should be cleaned up as soon as possible. If broken glass or other sharp objects are involved, care must be taken to ensure that the health care provider does not get cut. Body substance isolation is the rule when cleaning up spilled blood or OPIM.

Once appropriate personal protective equipment is donned, care should be taken to contain the spill. One way to achieve this is to cover the spill with paper towels. Once contained, the spill may be absorbed with additional paper towels and placed in a biohazard bag for disposal. A mixture of common household bleach (5.25% sodium hypochlorite diluted between 1:10 and 1:100 with water should be used to further disinfect the affected area.

When medical equipment becomes contaminated with blood and/or OPIM, it should be cleaned and disinfected before it is returned to service. OSHA recommends use of a bleach and water solution and/or a tuberculocidal disinfectant when decontaminating medical equipment or hard surfaces.

**ALERT**

Since hepatitis B can remain active for several days in dried blood, care must be taken even when cleaning up dried blood.

# PERSONAL HEALTH

**Personal health** is a three-part system that is a joint responsibility of both the employer and employee. This system includes physical examinations, vaccinations, and return to work authorizations.

## Physical Exams

Once hired, the employer must arrange for a **pre-entry physical exam** at no cost to the employee. This exam should screen for infectious disease, answer medical questions that would screen for pre-existing illnesses, and help to determine if the employee meets the **essential functions** of the position for which he/she has applied. Diagnostic tests for hepatitis B, tuberculosis, syphilis, and other diseases may be performed according to local needs. Many employers offer a battery of laboratory tests to assist the employee in identifying potential health problems. In recent years, many employers have offered memberships to health clubs, and some have placed fitness equipment in-house to encourage the personal fitness of their employees.

**ALERT**

The system of personal health may only be effective when it is comprehensive. Each of the three parts is required to provide maximum protection to the health care provider.

## Vaccinations

Immunizations against common infectious disease should be taken by all employees at risk of occupational exposure to blood and body fluid. The employee should ascertain that immunizations against tetanus, measles, mumps, and rubella are up to date. Boosters should be taken for any immunizations that are not current. A listing of vaccinations recommended for health care providers is shown in Figure 6-9.

| Immunization is Strongly Recommended | Immunization May Be Indicated |
|---|---|
| Hepatitis B | Hepatitis A |
| Influenza | Meningococcal Disease |
| Measles, Mumps, and Rubella | Pertussis |
| Varicella | Typhoid |
| | Smallpox (Vaccinia) |

FIGURE 6-9 Recommended immunizations for health care providers. (Source: Centers for Disease Control and Prevention.)

## Hepatitis B Vaccine

The Occupational Safety and Health Administration (OSHA) requires that employers offer the hepatitis B (HBV) vaccine free of charge to Category I employees who may be at risk of occupational exposure to blood and potentially infectious material. If the employee refuses the vaccine he/she must sign a standard declination form but may opt to take the vaccination at a later date, at the employer's expense.

The vaccination should be offered at a time and place convenient to the employee. Many employers allow employees to receive the vaccine while on duty. If the employee receives the vaccine while off duty, the employer may compensate the employee for time and/or travel expenses, if applicable. The intent of OSHA is that the employer must not make receiving the vaccine inconvenient for the employee.

The HBV vaccine is typically given in a series of three intramuscular injections. The first injection is given, followed by the second in one month. The third, and final, dose is given six months after the initial dose. Research has shown that immunity is best in young children (100% in ages 0–1) but is very good (average of 98%) in adults. Figure 6-10 graphically represents the chance for immunity after receiving the Recombivax HB hepatitis B vaccine.

| | | |
|---|---|---|
| Infants | 0–12 months | 100% |
| Children | 1–10 years | 99% |
| Adolescents | 11-20 years | 99% |
| Young Adults | 20–29 years | 98% |
| Adults | 20–39 years | 94% |
| Adults | over 40 years | 89% |

FIGURE 6-10 Immunity to hepatitis B after administration of Recombivax HB. (Source: Merck Vaccine Division. Recombivax HB is a registered trademark of Merck.)

Side effects of synthetic vaccines are minimal. The most common side effect is soreness at the injection site. Some people report flu-like symptoms that mimic the symptoms of the disease itself. Persons who are pregnant, nursing an infant, or are sensitive to yeast or its components should not receive the vaccine.

## Return to Work Authorization

An employee should be released by a physician to return to work after exposure to a communicable disease or after having been absent due to illness or injury. In some cases, the physician's discretion will allow the employee to return to work even while laboratory tests are pending. In a case where an employee is exposed to the blood or body fluid of a known HIV or HBV carrier, the employee may be reassigned to duty that does not include direct patient contact while awaiting the results of follow-up testing.

### ALERT

Some states have an *infected health care worker act* which requires health care providers to report if they become infected with a reportable disease.

Post exposure follow-up allows the employee to return to normal duty as soon as practical without exposing patients to undue risk. The employer must not terminate or demote an employee based on recommendations of a physician to limit the employee's activity to that which does not involve direct patient care. Even when employees return to work after having a cold or flu, the employer should have standard procedures for determining their ability to resume normal work duties.

## CONCLUSION

Personal health is an important responsibility shared by the employer and the employee. Both must know their roles and each must work with the other to assure safety for employees and patients, and to limit liability for the employer.

## CASE STUDY 6.1

Your patient is an elderly male who complains of chest wall pain and a productive cough with thick greenish/yellow sputum. He is receiving oxygen via face mask and must be suctioned occasionally.

REFLECT AND CONSIDER

➤ Which type of isolation would be appropriate for this patient?

➤ What personal protective equipment should be utilized in this situation?

## QUESTIONS FOR DISCUSSION

1. List at least four examples of common engineering controls.
2. List at least four examples of safe work practices.
3. Who is responsible for assuring that safe work practices are enforced?
4. Describe the differences in standard precautions and transmission-based precautions.
5. List and describe the three major types of transmission-based precautions.
6. Explain why body substance isolation (BSI) is generally the preferred method of isolation utilized by prehospital and out-of-hospital providers.
7. Who is responsible to launder or dispose of uniforms contaminated with blood or other potentially-infectious materials?
8. List and describe the three components of the personal health system.
9. List the contraindications of the hepatitis B vaccine.
10. Explain the procedure for cleaning up spilled blood.

## WORTH THINKING ABOUT

- What engineering controls at your agency/institution could be improved?
- Do you sometimes take shortcuts with safe work practices? What are the possible consequences of these shortcuts?
- What do you consider to be the most important safe work practice? Why?

## BIBLIOGRAPHY

Acello, B. (1998). *Patient care: Basic skills for the health care provider*. Albany, NY: Delmar.

Association for Professionals in Infection Control and Epidemiology. Web site. http://www.apic.org.

Centers for Disease Control and Prevention. (1998, May 15). Public health service guidelines for the management of health-care worker exposures to HIV and recommendations for postexposure prophylaxis. *Morbidity and Mortality Weekly Report 47*.

National Fire Academy. (1992). *Infection control for emergency response personnel: The supervisor's role*. Emmitsburg, MD: Author.

National Institute for Occupational Safety and Health. (1998). *Selecting, evaluating, and using sharps disposal containers*. Atlanta, GA: Author.

National Institute for Occupational Safety and Health. (1999). *Preventing needlestick injuries in health care settings*. Atlanta, GA: Author.

Offit, P. A., & Bell, L. M. (1999). *Vaccines: What every parent should know*. New York: IDG Books.

United States Air Force. Web site of the 74th Medical Group, Wright-Patterson Air Force Base.

United States Fire Administration. (1992). *Guide to developing and managing an emergency service infection control program*. Washington, DC: Author.

West, K. (2000, Spring). Personal safety solutions. *Emergency Products News*, 8–11.

# $\mathscr{C}$hapter 7
# Exposure Determination

▼ ▼ ▼ ▼ ▼ ▼ ▼

## $\mathscr{L}$EARNING OBJECTIVES

After completing this chapter, the reader should be able to:

- recognize a potential exposure to communicable disease.
- list six components normally required for an exposure to take place.
- discuss two questions health care providers may ask themselves to determine the likelihood of exposure to communicable disease.

## $\mathscr{K}$EY TERMS

- exposure
- method of travel
- portal of entry

## $\mathscr{I}$NTRODUCTION

Potential exposure to communicable disease can be a trying experience. This is why it is important for health care providers to understand what constitutes an exposure and what to do when a potential exposure occurs.

This chapter is not intended as a complete guide to exposure. It should, however, be helpful in determining if an exposure has occurred.

# CHAIN OF INFECTION

The chain of infection (Figure 7-1) illustrates six components necessary for communicable disease to be spread. A brief discussion of each follows.

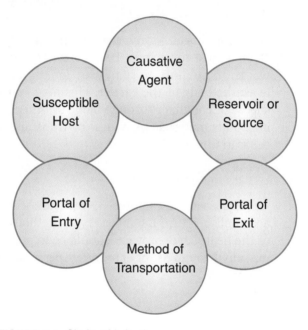

FIGURE 7-1  Chain of infection.

## Causative Agent

The causative agent of a disease is the virus, bacteria, fungus, rickettsia, or protozoan that causes the disease. For example, the causative agent of AIDS is the HIV virus and the causative agent of mononucleosis is the Epstein-Barr virus.

## Source or Reservoir

Each causative agent must have a place for the source to reside and grow, referred to as a *source* or *reservoir*. This is the person or object that carries the disease. In the case of rabies, the reservoir may be an infected dog. In tetanus, the source may be a rusty nail. It is important that health care providers isolate themselves from the source or potential reservoirs of infectious disease.

## Portal of Exit

For the pathogen to transfer from the carrier to a susceptible host there must be a portal of exit. In other words, there must be some way for the pathogen to leave the body of the carrier. This may be through a sneeze or cough, or through blood or other potentially infectious materials. A review of transmission methods is in Chapter 3.

## Mode of Transmission

As discussed in Chapter 3, transmission may be accomplished through a variety of methods. The goal of the health care provider should be to prevent transmission through use of appropriate personal protective equipment.

## Portal of Entry

For exposure to take place, the causative agent must find its way into the body of the exposed person. The way the pathogen enters the body is referred to as the portal of entry. Without a portal of entry, there is no exposure.

## Susceptible Host

The final requirement for exposure is a susceptible host. This means that the potentially exposed person must be susceptible to the disease. Health care providers may reduce their chance of susceptibility by maintaining a general state of health and being immunized against infectious diseases.

## &XPOSURE IN A NUTSHELL

Some of the components in the chain of infection may be difficult to measure. For that reason, a basic discussion of exposure follows. Though exposure is not as simple as the following definition, this section may be helpful to determine if a health care provider has been exposed to a communicable disease.

In simple terms, exposure to communicable disease requires two components. The first component is a method of travel or mode of transmission. A method of travel is the means through which the pathogen enters the body. In a needlestick incident, the needle is the method of travel. The infected material travels from the host patient to the employee by way of the needle. Common methods of travel are through needles and through direct contact with blood and/or body fluid.

The second component required in an exposure is the portal of entry. This is the path through which the infected material gains entry into the body. In a needlestick incident, the place where the needle punctures the skin is the portal of entry for the disease. Common portals of entry include punctures from needlesticks, non-intact or dry, cracked skin, and absorption through mucous membranes.

These two components should be considered when assessing the possibility of exposure. The absence of either factor is a good indication that no exposure took place. Figure 7-2 illustrates this point.

| Situation | Portal of Entry | Method of Travel | Exposure? |
|-----------|-----------------|------------------|-----------|
| Your glove tears and you get blood on your fingers. You have no cuts on your hands. | There is no portal of entry. | Yes, through the blood. | No, since there was no portal of entry. |
| Blood is splattered into your eye from a patient. | Yes, through the mucous membranes around the eyes. | Yes, through the blood. | Yes, there was a portal of entry and a method of travel. |

FIGURE 7-2 Exposure situations. This figure illustrates how both portal of entry and method of travel are important in assessing a possible exposure.

# AIRBORNE EXPOSURE

Exposure to airborne disease is often difficult to determine. An exposure occurs when droplets from a sneeze or cough are inhaled or deposited in an area of mucous membranes. These areas are highly vascular and may absorb contaminants into the bloodstream.

Exposure is also possible when an employee comes in contact with a patient in confined or close quarters. For this reason, persons who provide care to someone with an active airborne transmissible disease in close quarters, such as in the back of an ambulance, are considered to have been potentially exposed. Due to the proximity of the patient and the health care provider, exposure is assumed even if there is no definable exposure incident.

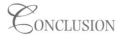

# CONCLUSION

When assessing a possible exposure, it is important to note both the portal of entry and the method of travel. If an employee believes he/she has been exposed, the incident should be reported to his/her supervisor as soon as practical. The supervisor should be trained and equipped to assist the employee in determining if an exposure took place, and in providing appropriate emergency care and documentation of the exposure incident. Chapter 8 covers what should be done once an exposure has occurred.

## CASE STUDY 7.1

You are caring for an adolescent who has sustained a head injury in a motor vehicle collision. He has no significant past medical history and takes no medications. While assisting in his care, he vomits on your arm. You are wearing gloves, but the gloves do not cover the area affected. Your skin is intact and your vaccinations are up to date.

### REFLECT AND CONSIDER

➤ Was there a method of travel?
➤ Was there a portal of entry?
➤ Have you been exposed? Why or why not?
➤ What actions should you take to further reduce your chance for exposure?

## QUESTIONS FOR DISCUSSION

1. Why is it harder to determine exposure to airborne transmitted diseases than exposure to bloodborne transmitted diseases?
2. What two things are necessary to prove an exposure occurred?
3. Why would someone who rides in an ambulance carrying a patient with an airborne communicable disease be considered to have been exposed? Would someone who rides in a car with that same person be considered exposed? Why or why not?

## WORTH THINKING ABOUT

- Consider what your first emotion might be after an exposure takes place.
- How can you assist a co-worker who has been exposed to blood or other potentially infectious material?

## BIBLIOGRAPHY

Acello, B. (1998). *Patient care: Basic skills for the health care provider*. Albany, NY: Delmar.

Centers for Disease Control and Prevention. (1989, June 23). Guidelines for prevention of transmission of human immunodeficiency virus and hepatis B virus to health-care and public safety workers. *Morbidity and Mortality Weekly Report 38* (S-6).

U.S. Department of Labor, Occupational Safety and Health Administration. (1991, Dec. 6). *Occupational exposure to bloodborne pathogens*. CFR 1910.1030, Final Rule.

U.S. Department of Labor, Occupational Safety and Health Administration. (1992). *Occupational exposure to bloodborne pathogens: Precautions for emergency responders*. OSHA 3130.

# Chapter 8
# Post Exposure

▼  ▼  ▼  ▼  ▼  ▼  ▼

## LEARNING OBJECTIVES

After completing this chapter, the reader should be able to:

- identify where written post-exposure protocols are found in his/her place of employment.
- list the steps that should be taken after an exposure.
- understand that confidential medical records must be maintained for exposure incidents.
- understand how to access outside assistance in dealing with post-exposure follow up.
- discuss why exposure may be stressful.
- list at least three ways to reduce stress.

## KEY TERMS

- exposure report form
- first aid
- post-exposure testing and follow up
- prophylaxis
- return-to-work authorization

# INTRODUCTION

Each employer should develop written protocols that guide employees through the exposure reporting process. These protocols are an integral part of the employer's exposure control plan and must be accessible to each employee who is at risk of occupational exposure. This chapter defines general guidelines for immediate response following an occupational exposure. Employees should become familiar with and follow protocols as published in the employer's exposure control plan.

# FIRST AID

The first priority following an exposure is to take immediate **first aid** measures. This includes bleeding control, wound cleansing and dressing, and/or flushing the eyes as appropriate. Other, more advanced first aid may be indicated and should be performed by appropriately trained personnel.

Simple wounds should be cleaned with soap and water. Dry, sterile dressings should be applied and held in place with sterile bandages. If the eyes are affected, they may be washed in a commercial eye wash station or with an improvised eye wash. (See Figure 8-1 for instructions.) If neither is available, the eyes should be washed with ordinary tap water for a minimum of twenty minutes.

# REPORTING

All exposures should be reported to the employee's immediate supervisor as soon as practical following an exposure incident. However, first aid measures take priority and should not be delayed in an attempt to notify the employee's supervisor.

## Improvised Eye Wash

*Items Needed:*

| 1 or more | bags of normal saline |
| 1 | nasal cannula |
| 1 | macrodrip IV tubing |

*TIP* : When flushing the eyes, encourage the patient to keep his/her eyes open and to alternately look in all directions. This will allow all exposed areas of the eyes and the surrounding membranes to be washed.

*Directions:*
Spike the bag of normal saline just as you would in preparation to start an IV.

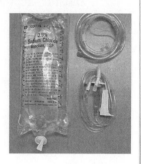

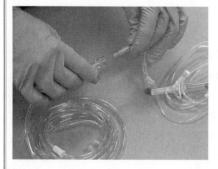

Attach the oxygen connector end of the nasal cannula to the distal end of the IV tubing.

Place patient in a supine or reclining position and place the prongs of the nasal cannula over the bridge of the nose so one prong is pointed toward each eye. Open the flow control valve on the IV tubing and adjust flow rate to keep a constant flood of saline in the eyes.

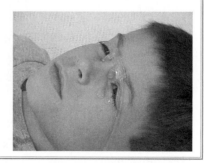

FIGURE 8-1 Eye wash instructions. This effective eye wash may be constructed with common items.

An **exposure report form** must be completed for each exposure and filed with the supervisor as directed in the employer's exposure control plan. The supervisor should then route the form to the designated officer who will assist the employee with **post-exposure testing and follow up**. Although medical records related to exposure are not kept in the employee's personnel record, exposure reports and medical follow-up records must be kept for the length of employment plus thirty years.

---

**National Clinicians' Post-Exposure Prophylaxis Hotline (PEPline)**

1-888-448-4911

24 hours a day

The PEPline was established to help clinicians counsel and treat health care providers who have occupational exposure to bloodborne diseases. It is staffed by physicians trained to give clinicians information, counseling and treatment recommendations for health care providers who have received needlestick injuries or other serious occupational exposure to bloodborne pathogens.

The PEPline is a service of the Centers for Disease Control and Prevention and the Health Resources and Services Administration in collaboration with the University of California, San Francisco and the San Francisco Department of Public Health.

---

FIGURE 8-2 National Clinician's Post-Exposure Prophylaxis Hotline (PEPline). (Source: Centers for Disease Control and Prevention.)

# ESTING

The designated officer will coordinate whatever testing and treatment is deemed necessary by the attending physician. The physician may test for HIV, HBV, and HCV or may prescribe medications as **prophylaxis** for other diseases (Figure 8-2). OSHA requires that the physician maintains all confidential medical records resulting from an exposure be maintained separately from employment records.

# OSHA REPORTING REQUIREMENTS

When an exposure incident meets one or more of the following criteria, the employer must record the incident as an injury on the OSHA 200 log (300 log after January 1, 2002). To be reportable to OSHA, the incident must:

- be work-related and involve a loss of consciousness, transfer to another job, or restriction of work or motion.
- be followed by a recommendation of medical treatment (including vaccinations or medication for prophylaxis).
- result in the diagnosis of seroconversion. Though seroconversion may have taken place, it should not be listed as such on the OSHA 200 (or 300) log.

It is generally accepted that employers who have ten or more employees at any time during the previous calendar year are required to maintain a log of occupational injuries and illnesses, though some variances may apply. These records must be kept for a minimum of five years after the accident and must be posted in the workplace each year.

## ALERT

 Since OSHA requires that some injuries (those involving fatalities or multiple hospitalizations) be reported regardless of the size of the company, the employer may want to consider voluntary compliance with OSHA reporting standards set forth in 29 CFR 1904.

## RETURN TO WORK

The **return to work authorization** may authorize an employee to return to normal job duties or it may limit the employee to duties that do not involve direct patient contact. The Americans with Disabilities Act (ADA) specifically names infectious disease as a disability that employers must not discriminate against. While it might be unwise to place a person with a known communicable disease in a setting of direct patient care, it would be discriminatory to terminate an individual based on a disability. Often, persons who are unable to return to duties involving direct patient care are reassigned in areas where exposure is less likely.

OSHA requires that the employer obtain and provide to the employee a copy of the physician's written opinion within 15 days of completion of the medical evaluation. The content of this report must include information that the employee has been informed of the results of the post-exposure evaluation and told about medical conditions resulting from the exposure incident which may require further evaluation and treatment. Any other findings must remain confidential and may not be contained in the written report.

## MANAGING STRESS

Even if no disease is contracted, exposure to communicable disease can be highly stressful to an individual, his/her spouse, significant other, and/or family. Employers should recognize the needs of employees and their families and provide appropriate counseling to help them cope with the stress of an exposure.

**ALERT**

Health care providers should be alert to signs of stress in their coworkers.

The offer of counseling by the employer is sometimes not enough. Health care providers have a responsibility to recognize their stress and the stress of their loved ones. Common signs and symptoms of stress include irritability, fatigue, lack of concentration, insomnia, and depression. See Figure 8-3 for a more comprehensive listing.

| Physical Changes | Emotional Changes |
|---|---|
| Headaches | Lack of concentration |
| Shortness of breath | Irritability |
| Increased pulse rate | Anger |
| Nausea | Mood swings |
| Insomnia | Over-reactive |
| Fatigue | Depression |
| Neck or back pain | Eating disorders |
| Dermatological problems | Anxiety |
| Chronic constipation/diarrhea | Low self-image |
|  | Hopeless feelings |

FIGURE 8-3 Physical and emotional signs of stress.

People choose to cope with stress in different ways. Before one may combat stress, however, its presence must first be recognized. Once this is accomplished, the health care provider may utilize a combination of counseling, education, and physical strategies to help reduce stress levels.

## Counseling

Counseling sessions with a mental health professional may help the health care provider and her family cope with the uncertainties of exposure. Participation in peer support groups and/or informal peer counseling may also prove helpful.

## Education

Learning more about the disease process may also help the health care provider cope with exposure. It is also important to educate the family of an exposed health care professional so they will understand the implications of exposure and the process of testing and follow up. OSHA requires that post-exposure counseling include recommendations for prevention of HIV including refraining from blood or organ donation, abstaining from sexual intercourse, and refraining from breast feeding infants during the follow-up period.

## Physical Strategies

While counseling and education deals with the psychological aspect of stress management, it is important that exposed health care providers utilize physical strategies that help reduce stress. This includes getting adequate rest, participation in leisure activities, and exercise. Physical exercise may relieve both muscle tension and mental tension, and may cause the release of endorphins, the body's own mood elevating chemicals.

Good nutrition is also essential to stress reduction and overall good health. For best results, health care providers should eat well balanced diets, limit their consumption of caffeine, and drink plenty of water each day.

Though many health care providers may find it hard to do so, they should also learn to relax. Many relaxation techniques are available, including breathing exercises, yoga, and meditation. Some people find relaxation in activities like gardening, fishing, golfing, or painting. Whether your idea of relaxation is resting in a hammock or running a marathon, it is important that you take the time to relax and rejuvenate your body, especially during times of extreme physical and/or emotional stress.

## CONCLUSION

While post-exposure reporting and medical follow up is an unpleasant chore at best, cooperation between the employer and the employee can make the process of testing and waiting more bearable. The health care providers can help themselves and their families by understanding the signs and symptoms of stress and utilizing strategies for stress reduction.

## CASE STUDY 8.1

You are caring for an elderly female patient when blood from a wound on her forehead is splattered in your eyes. You have no eye protection.

### REFLECT AND CONSIDER

> Is this considered an exposure? Why or why not?
> What is your first action?
> List, in order, the steps you would take to report this incident at your place of employment or school.

## QUESTIONS FOR DISCUSSION

1. How long must exposure records be kept by the employer?
2. What is the first priority after an exposure?
3. Can an employer fire an employee for contracting a communicable disease while off duty?
4. List at least five signs or symptoms of stress.
5. Discuss several strategies for stress reduction.

## WORTH THINKING ABOUT

- Consider the stress you and your loved ones might experience should you become exposed to a communicable disease.
- What is the most effective relaxation technique for you? What do other members of your family do for stress relief?

## BIBLIOGRAPHY

Acello, B. (1998). *Patient care: Basic skills for the health care provider.* Albany, NY: Delmar.

Colbert, B. J. (2000). *Workplace readiness for health occupations.* Albany, NY: Delmar.

Department of Health and Human Services. Web site. http://www.dhhs.gov.

National Fire Academy. (1992). *Infection control for emergency response personnel: The supervisor's role.* Emmitsburg, MD: Author.

United States Fire Administration. (1992). *Guide to developing and managing an emergency service infection control program.* Washington, DC: Author.

# $\mathcal{A}$ppendix A
## Answers to Questions for Discussion

▼   ▼   ▼   ▼   ▼   ▼   ▼

The answers provided are intended to stimulate further discussion and are not intended as a definitive answer to the questions presented. The answers should, however, assist the reader in understanding the concepts presented.

## $\mathcal{C}$HAPTER 1

1. What one disease has increased awareness of infection control the most in recent years?

   *Media coverage of AIDS has seemed to increase awareness of infection control over the past several years.*

2. What simple infection control procedure helped Dr. Ignaz Semmelweis save a number of lives in the 1800s?

   *The simple procedure of hand washing helped Dr. Semmelweis reduce the death rate due to infection at his hospital.*

3. List three pioneers in the field of infection control.

   *Ignaz Semmelweis proved that hand washing could prevent the spread of infection. Louis Pasteur's background in physics and chemistry led him to discover some of the basic principles of microbiology as we know it today. Joseph Lister applied Pasteur's principles and initiated the use of antiseptics.*

4. List at least three diseases that should concern health care workers today.

   *Many diseases should be of concern. Hepatitis C is certainly a threat to health care providers and should warrant concern. Other diseases such as hepatitis B, hepatitis non-ABC, HIV, and others should be of concern as well.*

## $\mathcal{C}$HAPTER 2

1. List three things required by OSHA regarding infection control.

   *OSHA mandates each employer with category I employees to develop an exposure control plan and offer hepatitis B vaccinations at no charge to the employee. Standards on personal protective equipment (PPE), record-keeping, training, and work practices were also developed by OSHA.*

2. If your state is not an OSHA state, why should you conform to OSHA regulations?

   *States that are not considered OSHA states must have a state plan that meets or exceeds OSHA standards.*

3. What is the intent of the Ryan White CARE Act?

   *The Ryan White Comprehensive AIDS Resources Emergency Act of 1990 gives employees the right to learn if they were exposed to infectious disease while caring for a patient.*

4. Explain routine notification.

   *Routine notification is where the hospital informs the health care provider who was potentially exposed to an airborne communicable disease.*

5. Explain notification by request.

   *Notification by request is where the health care provider requests to be notified of the source patient's seroconversion status after having been potentially exposed to the blood or OPIM of the patient.*

6. What is the role of the designated officer in an organization?

   *The designated officer serves as a liaison between the exposed health care provider and the hospital.*

# CHAPTER 3

1. Are all infectious diseases communicable? Explain your answer.

   *No. Some infectious diseases may not be considered person-to-person transmissible. For example, hanta virus is an infectious disease but it can not be transmitted person-to-person.*

2. Is a person more likely to become infected with HIV through direct or indirect contact? Explain your answer.

   *Since HIV is so weak outside the confines of the human body, indirect contact is highly unlikely.*

3. If you are exposed to a person with HIV today and have a negative blood test tomorrow, are you considered "safe?"

   *No. It may take weeks or months for a person to seroconvert and show a positive blood test. One negative test does not clear the person from infection.*

4. Name at least three ways diseases may be transmitted.

   *Diseases may be transmitted person-to-person through airborne, bloodborne, vector borne, or sexual transmission.*

5. List at least four causes of infectious disease.

   *Infectious disease may be caused by bacteria, viruses, fungi, rickettsia, or helminths.*

# CHAPTER 4

1. List and describe some of the key anatomical structures of the immune system?

   *The immune system is comprised of organs and structures from several organ systems including the integumentary, respiratory, gastrointestinal, and lymphatic systems. The tonsils protect the entrance of the respiratory system from invading pathogens. Lymph nodes filter harmful substances, and lymphatic vessels transport lymphatic fluid. The thymus produces T lymphocytes and the spleen serves as the site of development for monocytes and lymphocytes. The appendix is thought to help prevent disease by harboring nonpathogenic bacteria and the skin serves as a barrier that protects the body from invasion from external pathogens.*

2. Describe the process of phagocytosis and explain why it results in the production of pus.

   *Phagocytes attack and ingest invading pathogens by trapping them with arm-like projections and forming a sac around them. Once in the sac, pathogens are chemically destroyed. Phagocytes have a short life span. Once their job is done, phagocytes die and aggregate as pus, which is readily absorbed into the surrounding tissues.*

3. Which lasts longer, passive or active immunity? Why?

   *Active immunity lasts longer than passive immunity. Since the immunity is active, it means the body can produce antibodies to a certain antigen. This ability to produce antibodies makes active immunity longer acting than passive immunity, which is more immediate, but shorter acting.*

4. Of antigens and antibodies, which are more specific? Why?

   *Antibodies are more specific. Antigens mark cells as self or nonself. Antibodies are specific to only one antigen.*

5. List several signs and symptoms of infections. Discuss why these signs appear.

   *Characteristic signs of infection include hot, swollen, and reddened skin. These signs are caused by increased blood flow and vascular permeability in the affected area.*

# CHAPTER 5

1. Which infectious diseases should health care providers be most concerned with?

   *Health care providers should be concerned with any disease, though some may be of more concern than others. Though the availability of a vaccine has greatly reduced the incidence of hepatitis B, a threat to health care providers still exists. Hepatitis C has emerged as a major threat to health care providers and should warrant concern. Airborne communicable diseases like tuberculosis should also be a concern of health care providers since the possibility for transmission exists. Though these diseases are the ones that tend to get the most attention, any communicable disease, including influenza and pneumonia, should be a concern of health care providers.*

2. Experts have said it is 200 times easier to become infected with hepatitis B than with HIV. Why?

   *Hepatitis B is much more environmentally resistant than HIV.*

3. Why is it important to wear a mask when working in an area infested by rodents?

   *Hanta virus is spread through the inhalation of microscopic particles that contain rodent droppings or urine.*

4. Explain how the three types of lice are spread.

   *Head lice are spread through direct contact with an infested person or their personal items. Body lice are spread through indirect contact with personal belongings of an infested person. Crab lice are spread through sexual contact.*

5. Describe each of the four stages of syphilis.

   *Primary syphilis manifests itself through the development of a chancre ulcer. Secondary syphilis is noted by a skin rash that may include any part of the body but almost always involves the palms of the hands and the soles of the feet. This stage is a highly contagious stage. The third stage, latent syphilis, is a time when the syphilis is no longer contagious and may lie dormant for years. Tertiary syphilis, the fourth stage, can cause major complications and may last for years or decades.*

6. What infectious disease is sometimes referred to as lockjaw? Why?

   *Tetanus can cause muscular stiffness or paralysis in the neck and jaw, thus the name, lockjaw.*

7. Why is hepatitis C a serious threat to health care providers?

   *Since the symptoms of hepatitis C mimic those of influenza, hepatitis C poses a serious threat to health care providers who may not know they are infected until after serious liver damage has occurred.*

8. Why is legionellosis sometimes referred to as Legionaire's Disease?

*There was an outbreak at an American Legion convention in 1976 which resulted in the disease being referred to as Legionaire's Disease and the causative bacteria being renamed Legionella pneumophilia.*

# CHAPTER 6

1. List at least four examples of common engineering controls.

*Examples of engineering controls include the placement of sharps containers, eye wash stations, handwashing facilities, and storage of hazardous chemicals.*

2. List at least four examples of safe work practices.

*Safe work practices include hand washing, using personal protective equipment, not applying lip balm, and not smoking or eating in a work area.*

3. Who is responsible for assuring that safe work practices are enforced?

*While each employee should be responsible for safe work practices, enforcement is the responsibility of the employer.*

4. Describe the differences in standard precautions and transmission-based precautions.

*Standard precautions are used with all patients and advocate isolation from all body fluids (except sweat), non-intact skin, and mucous membranes. Transmission-based precautions are utilized for patients with a highly transmissible pathogen and may include airborne, droplet, or contact precautions.*

5. List and describe the three major types of transmission-based precautions.

*Airborne precautions are used with patients who are known or suspected to be infected with an airborne infectious disease. Emphasis is on respiratory protection and patient placement. Droplet precautions are used to protect from inhaling large particle droplets of moisture which carry contaminants. Isolation and respiratory protection is indicated. Contact precautions are used to protect against infection caused by coming in contact with an infected person or their personal items. Isolation from other patients is preferred and appropriate BSI is indicated.*

6. Explain why body substance isolation (BSI) is generally the preferred method of isolation utilized by pre-hospital and out-of-hospital providers.

*Body substance isolation contends that any body substance is potentially infectious and health care providers should isolate themselves from any potentially infectious substance. In areas where there is little control over the environment in which patient care takes place, this maximal protection helps protect health care providers from unexpected exposures.*

7. Who is responsible to launder or dispose of uniforms contaminated with blood or other potentially-infectious materials?

   *The responsibility for laundering or replacing uniforms is that of the employer.*

8. List and describe the three components of the personal health system.

   *A comprehensive system of personal health should include pre-entry physical examinations, vaccinations, and return to work authorizations.*

9. List the contraindications of the hepatitis B vaccine.

   *The hepatitis B vaccine should not be taken by those who are pregnant, nursing an infant, or are sensitive to yeast or any of its components.*

10. Explain the procedure for cleaning up spilled blood.

    *Once appropriate personal protective equipment is donned, care should be taken to contain the spill. One way to achieve this is to cover the spill with paper towels. Once contained, the spill may be absorbed with additional paper towels and placed in a biohazard bag for disposal. A mixture of common household bleach (sodium hypochlorite) and water should be used to further disinfect the affected area. The recommended mixture of bleach to water is between 1:10 to 1:100.*

# CHAPTER 7

1. Why is it harder to determine exposure to airborne transmitted diseases than exposure to bloodborne transmitted diseases?

   *The method of travel for bloodborne diseases is more apparent and easier to determine than that of airborne transmitted diseases. In essence, blood is easier to see than airborne droplets in a sneeze or cough.*

2. What two things are necessary to determine that an exposure occurred?

   *A method of travel and a portal of entry should be determined to indicate exposure.*

3. Why would someone who rides in an ambulance carrying a patient with an airborne communicable disease be considered

to have been exposed? Would someone who rides in a car with that same person be considered exposed? Why or why not?

*Persons who occupy a small space with someone with an airborne transmissible disease are, due to the close quarters, considered to have been exposed. This holds true both in an ambulance and in a car.*

# CHAPTER 8

1. How long must exposure records be kept by the employer?

   *Exposure records must be kept for the length of employment plus 30 years.*

2. What is the first priority after an exposure?

   *The first priority after an exposure should be immediate first aid treatment including cleansing wounds and controlling bleeding.*

3. Can an employer fire an employee for contracting a communicable disease while off duty?

   *To fire an employee for contracting a communicable disease would violate the provisions of the Americans with Disabilities Act which lists infectious disease as a disability. Job duties may be adjusted or medical leave may be granted depending on the situation and requirements of the job.*

4. List at least five signs or symptoms of stress.

   *Common signs and symptoms of stress include irritability, fatigue, lack of concentration, insomnia, and depression.*

5. Discuss several strategies for stress reduction.

   *People choose to cope with stress in different ways. Health care providers may choose to utilize a combination of counseling, education, and physical strategies to help reduce stress levels.*

# $\mathcal{A}$ppendix B
# Discussion of Case Studies

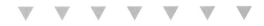

This appendix is intended to stimulate further thought and discussion of the cases in each chapter. It is not intended as an answer key, nor should it be construed as such. By learning what the instructor was thinking when the case studies were written, the reader will better appreciate the concepts presented.

## $\mathcal{C}$ASE 1.1

### OVERVIEW

This case is based on an actual case in which several teenagers at a cheerleading camp were exposed to *E. coli* after drinking contaminated water from an open ice barrel in the dormitory lobby. As mentioned in the case, campers reportedly dipped water bottles, hands, arms, and heads into the ice. Symptoms included nausea, vomiting, abdominal cramps, and bloody diarrhea.

### ANSWERS TO REFLECT AND CONSIDER

> What is the likely source of your patient's illness?

*The obvious contamination of the drinking water is a very likely source of illness. The likelihood of this being the source of illness is further reinforced since it can be determined that others who drank from the same barrel experienced similar symptoms.*

> How could this exposure have been prevented?

*Following basic infection control guidelines could have prevented this exposure. Drinking water should be kept in a closed container and, obviously, persons should not dip their heads, hands, etc. in it. Common sense and good housekeeping could have prevented this illness.*

> How could education have prevented this exposure?

*In this case the campers could have been educated to the possibility of cross contamination of the drinking water.*

## AUTHOR'S NOTES

- This case is based on an outbreak of *E. coli* in Texas in 1999. However, the symptoms of this illness may mimic those of several other conditions including amebiasis, salmonellosis, and shigellosis.
- Those of us who have children should educate them to the possibility of exposure to infectious disease and teach them strategies to protect them from disease.

ASE 2.1

### OVERVIEW

This case is fictitious, but is intended to illustrate the importance of conforming to national standards. Here, a hospital administrator decides to vary from national standards. If a suit is filed, the attorney may attempt to prove that negligence occurred as a result of the administrator's decision to vary from national standards.

### ANSWERS TO REFLECT AND CONSIDER

➤ Regardless of whether the hospital wins the suit, it may spend significant sums of money to defend the actions of the administrator. How can hospital administration prevent such lawsuits from occurring in the future?

*The easiest way to prevent lawsuits such as this is to adhere to national standards.*

### AUTHOR'S NOTE

- When an agency like the Centers for Disease Control and Prevention establishes standards, health care providers should take care to follow their guidelines.

ASE 3.1

### OVERVIEW

This case conveys the story of a friendly influenza virus named Flo who tells the tale of how she has moved from one host to another. The virus was spread through the sneeze of the mail carrier and passed on to the secretary who carried the mail, and the virus, to

Mr. West. After picking up the germs on his hands, Mr. West spread the virus to the surface of the water cooler. He also passed the virus to the foreman who spread it to Mrs. Cooper who, in turn, spread the virus to a shopping cart handle. The virus was then spread to Billy, a two-year-old, who chewed on the shopping cart handle.

## ANSWERS TO REFLECT AND CONSIDER

> What one simple procedure could have prevented this spread of infection from happening?

*Though the spread of this virus could have been stopped at several points within this case study, the simple procedure of hand washing at any point could have prevented the spread of the virus.*

> Discuss how many opportunities there were to stop the passage of the virus.

*It is nearly impossible to name every opportunity to stop the virus as hand washing at nearly any time during the scenario could have stopped the spread. Unfortunately, once the virus was spread on the mail, the virus went in several different directions.*

> List several ways viruses like influenza are spread.

*Influenza may be spread through droplets in a sneeze or cough. These droplets may be directly inhaled or deposited in mucous membranes around the mouth, nose, or eyes. The virus may be spread indirectly through contact with contaminated surfaces or objects.*

## AUTHOR'S NOTE

- This case illustrates the importance of hand washing and the everyday practice of infection control. An article in the August, 2000 issue of *Emergency Medical Services* suggests that health care providers who routinely wash their hands are much less likely to be sick than those who do not often wash their hands.

# CASE 4.1

## OVERVIEW

This case illustrates the story of how phagocytosis works with a little help from Luke (a leukocyte), Mac (a macrophage), and Newt (a neutrophil). It relates how the group (known collectively as phagocytes) is summoned to an area of pathogen invasion by chemotaxis. Luke goes on to explain how the process of phagocytosis works.

## ANSWERS TO REFLECT AND CONSIDER

> Why does someone with an infection have a high white blood cell (WBC) count?

*When an infection invades the body, white blood cells (or leukocytes) are summoned to the scene by chemotaxis. This need for additional white blood cells results in increased production which increases the white cell count.*

> Which is the earlier sign of infection: hot, red skin or the presence of pus?

*Hot red skin is the earlier sign which indicates increased blood flow due to the arrival of phagocytes. Pus results from the death of phagocytes, which comes within one or two days.*

## AUTHOR'S NOTE

- An understanding of how the body protects itself from infectious disease can help protect the health care provider against infectious disease and better understand the patient's reaction to the disease process.

ASE 5.1

## OVERVIEW

This study outlines the case of a 46-year-old male who complains of fever, bloody diarrhea, abdominal cramps, and vomiting over a two-day period. The patient works in the poultry industry and has regular contact with young fowl. This case is based on an actual cluster of 40 patients in Missouri, who, during a period of two months in 1999, complained of symptoms similar to those used in this case. Ninety-two percent (92%) of those involved reported exposure to young fowl just prior to the episode.

## ANSWERS TO REFLECT AND CONSIDER

> Based on the patient's occupation, what is the most likely source of his illness?

*Since salmonella can be spread through raw poultry, a case of salmonellosis may be expected.*

> What other illnesses are his signs and symptoms consistent with?

*The symptoms in this case are consistent with several other diseases and conditions which affect the gastrointestinal system including gastroenteritis, amebiasis, E coli, and shigellosis.*

➤ What precautions would you take when treating this patient?

*Standard precautions and thorough hand washing are in order, as for any patient.*

## AUTHOR'S NOTES

- Though salmonellosis is considered a foodborne illness it may be spread through contact with young fowl and reptiles. Patients exhibiting symptoms consistent with salmonellosis should be questioned about contact with these animals, and asked whether they have ingested any unpasteurized dairy products, undercooked poultry, or eggs that may have been contaminated.

- The CDC reports that, although most of the 1.4 million cases of salmonellosis that occur each year in the United States are caused by foodborne causes, direct contact with animals, usually young birds and reptiles, may also be a source of infection.

# CASE STUDY 5.2

## OVERVIEW

This case is based on an actual incident in April, 2000 in which a 33-year-old female had been out of state for a week and presented to the hospital upon return with a rash, fever, cough, and small white punctate lesions on the buccal mucosa.

## ANSWERS TO REFLECT AND CONSIDER

➤ What is the likely diagnosis for this patient?

*Based on the progression of signs and symptoms for this patient, measles should be expected.*

➤ What questions would you ask the patient about her past medical history?

*It would be appropriate to ask the patient about her immunization status.*

➤ How could her disease be transmitted? What precautions should you take?

*Measles can be spread by direct contact with nasal or throat secretions of infected persons or by airborne transmission. The health care provider should use standard precautions including a mask. If the patient can tolerate a mask, one may be placed for additional protection.*

➤ Would you have taken the same precautions had the patient presented four days ago with nausea, headache, fever and body ache? Why or why not?

*Though the patient's symptoms had not progressed to the second phase of measles at that time, the same precautions should have been taken. By utilizing maximal, rather than minimal, protection the health care provider reduces the opportunity for occupational exposure.*

## AUTHOR'S NOTES

- Health care providers should be immunized for all the normal childhood diseases in an effort to protect them and their patients.
- Since adults sometimes get childhood diseases, health care providers should be cognizant of that possibility.

 ASE 6.1

## OVERVIEW

In this case your patient is an elderly male who complains of chest wall pain and a productive cough. Thick greenish/yellow sputum is present. Oxygen is being administered by face mask and he must be suctioned occasionally.

## ANSWERS TO REFLECT AND CONSIDER

➤ Which type of isolation would be appropriate for this patient?

*Standard precautions or body substance isolation should be utilized to avoid contact with the sputum or any droplets contained in the cough.*

➤ What personal protective equipment should be utilized in this situation?

*Gloves are indicated since suctioning is necessary. Since the patient is coughing, a mask and eye protection are indicated. Since there is possibility of splash, a gown should also be indicated.*

## AUTHOR'S NOTES

- The recommendation is that the use of personal protective equipment be maximal, rather than minimal, in any case, but especially in cases where airborne transmission is possible.
- When suctioning, take care to protect your uniform from splashes and remember to wash your hands after each contact.

 ASE 7.1

## OVERVIEW

In this scenario, a head-injured patient vomits on your arm. You are wearing gloves, but the gloves do not cover the affected area. Your skin is intact and your vaccinations are up-to-date. The goal of this case is to determine if there has been an exposure.

## ANSWERS TO REFLECT AND CONSIDER

➤ Was there a method of travel?

*Yes. The vomit may carry infectious disease.*

➤ Was there a portal of entry?

*No. Since your skin is intact there is no place for the disease to enter the body. If there was an open sore or cut on your arm there would have been an exposure.*

➤ Have you been exposed? Why or why not?

*No. Since there was no portal of entry it is unlikely that an exposure has occurred.*

➤ What actions should you take to further reduce your chance for exposure?

*You should wash your hands and arms at your earliest opportunity and take care not to splash the vomit in your eyes or face.*

## AUTHOR'S NOTES

- Though exposure is a complicated process the health care provider may ask two simple questions to establish the likelihood of exposure. 1) Was there a method of travel? 2) Was there a portal of entry? If both of these questions are answered in the affirmative, it is likely that the health care provider has been exposed.
- If in doubt about an exposure, ask your supervisor or designated officer for direction. Health care providers should utilize all available resources to determine their exposure status.

ASE 8.1

## OVERVIEW

This case presents a situation where blood is splattered in your eyes. Beyond that, the details are not very important. For this reason, they were omitted.

## ANSWERS TO REFLECT AND CONSIDER

> Is this considered an exposure? Why or why not?

*This is an exposure. There is a method of travel (through the blood) and a portal of entry (through the mucous membranes around the eyes). The combination suggests an exposure.*

> What is your first action?

*The first action should be to wash the blood from your eyes. This should be accomplished with a commercial eye wash or with an improvised eye wash described in Figure 8-1.*

> List, in order, the steps you would take to report this incident at your place of employment or school.

*While specific protocols may vary by agency, general steps to reporting include immediate first aid, reporting the incident to your immediate supervisor, and a medical examination.*

## AUTHOR'S NOTES

• Health care providers should be aware of the post exposure protocols for their agency.

• It is important to take exposure seriously, regardless of the age and expected seroconversion status.

## BIBLIOGRAPHY

Centers for Disease Control and Prevention. (2000, April 14). Salmonellosis associated with chicks and ducklings—Michigan and Missouri, Spring, 1999. *Morbidity and Mortality Weekly Report 49* (14).

Centers for Disease Control and Prevention. (2000, April 21). *Escherichia coli* 0111:H8 outbreak among teenage campers—Texas, 1999. *Morbidity and Mortality Weekly Report 49* (15).

Dernocoeur, K. (2000, August). *Soap for safety. Emergency Medical Services.* p. 28.

# Appendix C
## Glossary

▼   ▼   ▼   ▼   ▼   ▼   ▼

**acquired immunity**—type of specific immunity that one is not born with. May be artificial (caused by immunization) or natural (resulting from nondeliberate exposure to antigens after birth).

**acquired immunodeficiency syndrome (AIDS)**—fatal illness caused by infection with the Human Immunodeficiency Virus (HIV).

**active immunity**—refers to an individual who has the ability to produce antibodies to a certain antigen.

**adsorb**—to attract and retain another material.

**airborne transmission**—refers to the transmission of microorganisms spread by a cough or sneeze.

**airborne precautions**—isolation method for patients known or suspected to be infected with airborne transmissible diseases, where emphasis is placed on patient placement and respiratory protection.

**Americans with Disabilities Act (ADA)**—legislation designed to prohibit discrimination against persons with disabilities. "Contagious disease" is specifically listed as a qualifying disability.

**antibodies**—proteins that attach themselves to antigens to mark them for destruction.

**antigens**—chemical markers that identify cells as self (human) or nonself (foreign).

**antiviral**—pertains to something that opposes, interferes with replication of, or weakens the action of a virus.

**aphasia**—loss of the ability to speak.

**asymptomatic**—without symptoms or complaint.

**attenuated**—thinned, reduced, or weakened.

**autoimmune response**—cells or antibodies created by and working against the body's own tissues.

**bacteria**—a type of living microorganism that can produce disease in a host. Bacteria can self-produce and some produce toxins that are harmful to their host.

**B lymphocytes**—white blood cells primarily responsible for humoral immunity.

**basophils**—phagocytic leukocytes similar in form and function to mast cells.

**Bell's Palsy**—unilateral paralysis of facial muscles caused by dysfunction of the seventh cranial nerve.

**biohazard container**—a puncture-resistant container used for the proper disposal of contaminated needles and other contaminated items.

**bloodborne transmission**—pertains to the spread of microorganisms present in human blood that are capable of causing disease.

**body substance isolation (BSI)**—the school of thought regarding personal protective equipment regards any substance related to the body as infectious, and advocates placing a barrier between the employee and the substance.

**breach of duty**—failure to meet the obligation of providing care.

**cancerous**—pertaining to a malignant neoplasm.

**casual contact**—everyday contact with those who live, work, or go to school together. *See also* household contact.

**category I employee**—an OSHA term that refers to an employee who is considered at the greatest risk of occupational exposure to communicable disease.

**causative agent**—an agent that causes a particular disease.

**cell-mediated immunity**—immunity provided by T cells.

**Centers for Disease Control and Prevention (CDC)**—division of the U.S. Department of Health and Human Services that conducts ongoing research on infection control issues.

**chancre**—the primary sore or lesion of syphillis.

**chemotaxis**—movement in response to chemical stimulation.

**civil liability**—a wrong against another individual for which remedy damages are awarded. Typically in infection control issues the liability is a result of not meeting an established standard.

**communicable disease**—an infectious disease that can be transmitted from one person to another.

**complement proteins**—group of approximately 20 inactivated plasma proteins, called *complement*, which circulate in the blood. When activated, complement proteins cause rupture of the cell that triggered it.

**congenital rubella syndrome (CRS)**—high incidence of congenital birth defects resulting from maternal infection with rubella during the first trimester.

**conjuctivitis**—inflammation of the membrane lining of the eyelids, and covering the eyeball.

contact precautions—CDC guidelines for limiting contact with an infected person or his/her personal items.

damages—monetary or other loss.

debridement—removal of dead tissue or foreign matter from a wound.

designated officer—required by the Ryan White CARE Act of 1990. This person is a liaison between the employee and the physician or hospital when an exposure takes place.

direct transmission—transmission of a disease from one person to another through direct contact with infected blood, body fluids, or other infectious material.

disseminated intravascular coagulation (DIC)—hemorrhagic syndrome that occurs following an uncontrolled activation of clotting factors.

dormant—inactive.

droplet precautions—CDC guidelines intended to protect the health care provider from inhaling large particle droplets of moisture carrying contaminants.

duty to act—refers to the duty of a caregiver to provide appropriate medical care.

dysuria—difficulty or pain in urination.

encephalitis—inflammation of the brain.

engineering controls—actions taken by the employer to make the workplace safer by engineering safety directly into the workplace.

enteric—referring to the intestine.

enterohemorrhagic—refers to bleeding within or from the intestines.

environmentally resistant—durable or able to survive outside the confines of the human body.

epididymitis—inflammation of the epididymis.

essential functions—actions or attributes the employee must meet, with or without accommodation, to fulfill the duties of a job.

exposure—contact with blood, body fluids, or potentially infectious material.

exposure control plan—written document required by OSHA that outlines the employer's infection control plan.

exposure report form—standard form used by an employee to report an occupational exposure.

exudates—fluid that seeps out of a tissue or its capillaries, usually due to injury or inflammation.

first aid—general measures taken in the minutes after an accident or illness that might include such actions as bleeding control and cleaning wounds.

fungus—plantlike organism that may grow as single cells (e.g., yeast) or as multicellular colonies (e.g., mold).

Gullain-Barre Syndrome—acute, progressive disease that affects the spinal nerves.

helminths—parasitic worms.

helper T cells—specialized T cells that have a receptor for immunoglobulin M antibodies.

hemolytic uremic syndrome—hemolytic anemia and thrombocytopenia occurring with acute renal failure. Associated with infection, complications of pregnancy following normal delivery, or oral contraceptive use.

hepatitis B virus (HBV)—a bloodborne virus that poses a serious threat to employees at risk to occupational exposure. The hepatitis B virus is very dangerous because it can stay active outside the body for long periods of time.

hepatitis C virus (HCV)—virus that affects the liver. Currently the most common chronic bloodborne infection in the U.S.

high efficiency particulate air (HEPA) respirator—respirator approved for employees exposed to patients to tuberculosis.

household contact—everyday contact with those who live, work, or go to school together. *See also* casual contact.

humoral immunity—type of specific immunity that occurs within plasma. Also called antibody-mediated immunity.

incubation period—the time from the exposure to a disease until the first appearance of symptoms.

indirect transmission—transmission of a disease from one person to another without direct contact.

infectious disease—a disease that results from an invasion of a host from a disease producing organism. This organism may be in the form of a virus, bacteria, fungus, or parasite.

inflammatory response—second line of protection against pathogens. The inflammatory response utilizes specialized leukocytes, called neutrophils and macrophages, to find and destroy invading pathogens through a process called phagocytosis.

inherited immunity—specific immunity that is acquired in utero.

**integumentary system**—the skin and its structures.

**interferon**—a protein that defends against viral infections. By inhibiting the ability of a virus to cause a disease, interferon prevents viruses from replicating in cells.

**killer T cells**—lymphocytes able to recognize, bind to, and kill antigens located on the surface of pathogenic cells. By releasing lymphotoxin, a powerful poison, killer T cells eliminate pathogens directly.

**Koplik's spots**—distinctive, small, irregular, red spots with a bluish or white speck in the center. Found on the buccal and lingual mucosa during early stages of measles. Often a tell-tale sign of measles.

**lacrimation**—secretion of tears.

**lesion**—pathologic change in the tissues, which may be benign or malignant.

**leukocytes**—white blood cells whose function is to protect the body against pathogens.

**lymphocytes**—type of leukocyte formed in bone marrow. Lymphocytes participate in immunity.

**lymphotoxins**—toxin from T lymphocytes that damage many cell types.

**lysozyme**—enzyme destructive to cell walls of certain bacteria.

**macrophage**—type of phagocyte that migrates out of the bloodstream and grows to several times its original size. Found in the alveoli, lymph nodes, brain, liver, and spleen, macrophages ingest invading and dead cells.

**Mantoux test**—diagnostic test for tuberculosis that involves the intradermal injection of tuberculin bacteria particles.

**mast cells**—found in all tissues of the body, mast cells play a role in the inflammatory process.

**method of travel**—the means through which pathogens enter the body.

**mite**—transparent or semi-transparent arthropod, which may be parasitic on man or animals, causing skin irritations.

**mitotic**—relating to the process of reproduction of cells caused by indirect cell division.

**myalgia**—muscle pain.

**myoclomus**—referring to one or a series of shock-like contractions of a muscle group, caused by a central nervous system lesion.

**National Fire Academy (NFA)**—an organization responsible for much of the early training materials developed for infection control.

**National Fire Protection Association (NFPA)**—an organization that set landmark standards for the prevention of infection diseases.

**natural killer cells**—type of lymphocyte that recognizes and destroys infected or tumor cells. Natural killer cells do not have to be activated by an external antigen, so they are considered non-specific.

**necrosis**—pertaining to cell death.

**negligence**—act of being neglectful, or not acting as a health care provider of similar experience and training would.

**neutrophils**—the most numerous of the phagocytes, neutrophils are mature white blood cells that ingest the microorganisms through phagocytosis and die within one or two days.

**nonsteroidal anti-inflammatory drugs (NSAIDs)**—group of over-the-counter medications commonly used to reduce swelling.

**nosocomial infections**—infection originating in a hospital.

**notification by request**—made by any employee who is potentially exposed to a communicable disease while providing patient care.

**nuchal rigidity**—stiffness of the neck.

**nymph**—developmental stage in certain arthropods, resembling an adult.

**occupational exposure**—exposure of an employee to communicable disease while performing job-related duties.

**Occupational Safety and Health Administration (OSHA)**—an organization charged with the protection of employees in the workplace.

**oocyst**—dormant form of cryptosporidium; a parasitic protozoan that lives in the intestines of people and animals.

**other potentially infectious material (OPIM)**—material, other than blood, that may reasonably be expected to be infectious.

**parasitic**—referring to organisms that live in or on the body of the host, and gains some advantage from the host.

**paresthesia**—abnormal sensation (burning, prickling, etc.) for no apparent reason.

**passive immunity**—refers to immunity from an outside source or transferred to someone who was not previously immune. Passive immunity provides temporary, but immediate, protection.

**pathogenic**—causing disease or abnormality.

**pediculicide**—agent used to destroy lice.

**pelvic inflammatory disease (PID)**—inflammation of some or all of the pelvic reproductive organs.

**peripheral neuropathy**—disorder affecting the peripheral or autonomic nervous system.

**personal health**—a three-part plan consisting of physical examinations, vaccinations, and authorization to return to duty or work.

**personal protective equipment**—any equipment used to protect the employee from occupational exposure to blood and body fluid.

**petechial rash**—rash marked by small hemorrhages within the skin.

**phagocytosis**—inflammatory process in which phagocytes (cells capable of phagocytosis) attack and ingest the invading agent.

**photophobia**—abnormal intolerance to light.

**portal of entry**—path through which pathogens gain entry into the body.

**post-exposure testing and follow up**—a series of laboratory tests and medical exams that are performed after an exposure incident.

**pre-entry physical exam**—exam required before entry into service.

**prodromal**—early symptom of a disease.

**prophylaxis**—preventative treatment.

**prostatitis**—inflammation of the prostate.

**protozoans**—the simplest organisms in the animal kingdom. Many are single-celled, though some colonize.

**proximate cause**—relation between an inappropriate action or inaction and damages. To prove negligence one must show that a breach of duty caused damages.

**purulent**—containing or consisting of pus.

**replicate**—to duplicate or reproduce.

**return to work authorization**—medical approval to return to work/duty after an exposure incident or any illness requiring the employee to miss work for medical reasons.

**rickettsia**—parasitical bacteria that depend on living cells for growth.

**routine notification**—provided by the treating facility or hospital to employees who are exposed to a patient found to have an airborne communicable disease.

**Ryan White Comprehensive Aids Resources Emergency (CARE) Act of 1990**—landmark legislation that gives employees the right to learn if they were exposed to infectious disease in the course of caring for a patient.

**safe work practices**—rules of conduct, set forth by an employer's standard operating procedure or employee handbook, governing practices and procedures that make the workplace safer.

**saprophytic**—referring to an organism that grows on dead organic matter.

sebum—oily substance secreted by the sebaceous glands.

septic arthritis—acute inflammation of synovial membranes caused by bacterial infection.

seroconversion—a change in the status of a person's serum test.

sexual transmission—the passing of a disease through any type of sexual contact.

sexually transmitted disease (STD)—disease transmitted through sexual contact.

sharps containers—puncture-resistant and leak-proof biohazard container intended for discarded needles, scalpels, and other sharps.

specific immunity—immunity against specific foreign pathogens.

standard of care—level of care expected of a given level of health care provider. A basis for comparison.

Standard precautions—CDC recommendations that apply to all patients receiving care in hospitals. These precautions apply to contact with blood, all body fluids (with the exception of sweat), nonintact skin, and mucous membranes.

susceptible—at risk of infection.

systemic bacteremia—presence of bacteria in circulating blood.


T lymphocytes—specialized lymphocytes that develop in the thymus, and typically reside in the spleen and lymph nodes; responsible for cell-mediated immunity.

T suppressor cells—specialized lymphocytes that regulate the function of B cells and other T cells.

therapeutic—related to curing or treating a disease or condition.

thrombocytopaenia—condition of having an abnormally small number of platelets in the circulating blood.

transmission-based precautions—CDC recommendations utilized with those patients known or suspected to be infected with highly transmissible or epidemiologically important pathogens. One or more of three types of transmission-based precautions may be used, depending on the way a given disease is transmitted.

tuberculosis—a lower respiratory tract infection that is spread through airborne water droplets.

tumor—a new growth of tissue in which cell multiplication is uncontrolled.


urethral strictures—lesion that reduces the inside diameter of the urethra, typically caused by inflammation.

**vector borne transmission**—transmission of a disease-causing organism through an outside source, or a vector.

**virulence**—degree of pathogenicity of a microorganism.

**virus**—microorganism that resides within other living cells and cannot reproduce outside a living cell.

**window phase**—time of exposure to a disease until a serum test reads "positive."

# Index

**Note:** Page numbers in **bold type** refer to information contained in figures

Acquired immunity, defined, 42
Acquired immunodeficiency syndrome (AIDS), 3
    overview of, 52–53
Active immunity, defined, 43
Acyclovir, 73
    herpes simplex and, 73, 74
ADA (Americans with Disabilities Act), 14
Adenoids, 35
Adsorbed vaccine (RVA), 92
AIDS (Acquired immunodeficiency syndrome), 3
    overview of, 52–53
Airborne exposure, 138
Airborne precautions, communicable disease, 121
Airborne transmission of disease, 26
Allergic reactions, Immunoglobulin E (IgE) and, 44
Amebiasis, overview of, 54
Americans with Disabilities Act (ADA), 14
Anthrax, overview of, 55–56
Antibodies, defined, 43–44
Antibody-mediated immunity, 45
Antigens, defined, 43
Appendix, vermiform, 36–37
Association for Professionals in Infection Control and Epidemiology, 117
Atrioventricular block, 81
Augmentin, pneumonia and, 90
Autoimmune disorders, body systems affected by, **38**
Autoimmune rejection, defined, 38

B lymphocytes, described, 44–45
Bacteria, defined, 24
Basophils, Immunoglobulin E (IgE) and, 44
Bell's palsy, Lyme disease and, 81

Biohazard containers, communicable disease and, 113–114
Biological weapons, Anthrax as, 56–57
Bleach, 127
Bloodborne transmission of disease, 26
Body louse, 77
Body system affected *See* specific disease
Bone marrow, immune system and, 37
*Bordetella pertussis*, 87
*Borrelia burgdorferi*, 81
Botulism, overview of, 56–57
Breach of duty, described, 17

Case studies, 158–165
Casual contact, disease transmission and, 27
Category I employees, 11
Causative agent
    defined, 51, 135
    *see also* specific disease
CDC (Centers for Disease Control and Prevention)
    infection control and, 15–16
    percutaneous injuries estimated by, 14–15
Ceftriaxone, meningococcal meningitis and, 84
Cell-mediated immunity, 45
Centers for Disease Control and Prevention (CDC)
    infection control and, 15–16
    percutaneous injuries estimated by, 14–15
Cephalosporin, pneumonia and, 90
Chancre ulcer, 102
Chemotaxis, inflammatory response and, 40
Chickenpox, overview of, 58–60
Chlamydia, overview of, 57–58
*Chlamydia trachomatis*, 57–58
Chloramphenicol, Rocky Mountain Spotted Fever and, 93
Ciprofloxacin, meningococcal meningitis and, 84
Civil liability, described, 16–17
Clean-up, communicable disease and, 127
Clostridium botulinum, 56
*Clostridium tetani*, 103
CMV (Cytomegalovirus), overview of, 62–63
Communicable disease
    biohazard containers and, 113–4
    clean-up and, 127
    defined, 23

engineering controls and, 112–116
eye protection and, 124–125
eye wash stations and, 116
gloves and, 123–4
gowns and, 126
handling/using sharps and, 118–120
handwashing and, 113
HEPA respirators and, 124
versus infectious disease, **24**
laundering and, 126
masks/respirators and, 124
medical devices and, 114–5
protection from, 111–131
safe work practices and, 116–122
uniforms and, 126
Communicable period, defined, **29**
Community health, 17–18
Complement proteins, 42
Congenital rubella syndrome (CRS), 95
Conjunctivitis, Chlamydia and, 58
Contact precautions, communicable disease, 122
Counseling, post exposure, 148
Crab louse, 77
Crohn's disease, **38**
Crotamiton, scabies and, 99
CRS (Congenital rubella syndrome), 95
Cryptosporidiosis, overview of, 60–62
Cryptosporidium, 60
Cytomegalovirus (CMV), overview of, 62–63

Damages, described, 17
Decontamination, 127
Designated officer, Ryan White care act and, 14
Dhboie itch, 25
Diabetes mellitus, type 1, **38**
Direct exposure, 23–24
Discussion questions, test review, 151–157
Disease
    cause of, 24–25
    infectious/communicable, defined, 23
    transmission of, 26–27
Disease period, defined, **29**
Disinfection, 127

Disseminated intravascular coagulation (DIC), rabies and, 92
Doxycycline
    pneumonia and, 90
    syphilis and, 103
DPT vaccine, pertussis and, 88
Droplet precautions, communicable disease, 122
DtaP vaccine, pertussis and, 88
Duty to act, described, 17
Dysentery, 25
Dysuria, Chlamydia and, 58

### E

E. coli, overview of, 64–65
Education, post exposure, 148
Encephalitis, rubella and, 95
Engerix B, 69–70
Engineering controls, communicable disease and, 112–116
*Entamoeba histolytica*, 54
Enterohemorrhagic group, 64
Enzymes, nonspecific immunity and, 39
Epididymitis, gonorrhea and, 65
Epstein-Barr virus, 85–86
Erythrocytes, immune system and, 37
Erythromycin
    pertussis and, 88
    pneumonia and, 90
    syphilis and, 103
Escherichia coli, overview of, 64–65
Ethambutol, tuberculosis and, 106
Exposure
    airborne transmission, 138
    described, 137–138
    post. *see* Post exposure
    situations, **138**
    types of, 23–24
Exposure control plan, 11
    contents, **12**
Exposure determination, 134–139
Exposure report form, 144
Eye protection, communicable disease and, 124–125
Eye wash
    improvised, **143**
    instructions, **143**
    stations, communicable disease and, 116

First aid, post exposure, 142
Foscarnet, CMV (Cytomegalovirus) and, 63
Fungus, defined, 25

Ganciclovir, CMV (Cytomegalovirus) and, 63
Gastric acids, nonspecific immunity and, 39
Genital herpes, 26, 74–75
Germ theory, Louis Pasteur and, 2
German measles, overview of, 94–97
Glossary, 166–174
Gloves, communicable disease and, 123–4
Gonorrhea, 26
    overview of, 65–66
Gowns, communicable disease and, 126
Graves' disease, 38
Gullain-Barre syndrome, rubella and, 95

*H. influenzae*, 89
Hand washing
    communicable disease and, 113
    Ignaz Semmelweis and, 2
    importance of, 117–118
    technique, **119**
    tips, **117**
Hantavirus pulmonary syndrome, overview of, 66–67
Hard measles, overview of, 82–83
Hashimoto's thyroiditis, **38**
HBV (Hepatitis B), 4–5
    overview of, 69–70
HCV (Hepatitis C), 4–5
    overview of, 70–72
HDCV (Human diploid cell vaccine), 92
Head louse, 77
    detail of, **78**
Health care providers *See* specific disease
Health care workers
    infected, 5–7
        with HIV, **6**
        secondary to occupational exposure, **6**

Helminths, defined, 25
Helper T cells, 45
Hemolytic uremic syndrome, 64
HEPA respirators, communicable disease and, 124
Hepatitis A, overview of, 68–69
Hepatitis B (HBV), 4–5
    immunity to, **130**
    overview of, 69–70
    vaccine, 129–130
Hepatitis C (HCV), 4–5
    overview of, 70–72
Hepatitis D (delta), overview of, 72–73
Hepatitis E, overview of, 72–73
Hepatitis G, overview of, 72–73
Hepatitis non-ABC, overview of, 72–73
Herpes simplex 1, overview of, 73–74
Herpes simplex 2, overview of, 74–75
Herpesvirus group, CMV (Cytomegalovirus) and, 62
Histamine response, Immunoglobulin E (IgE) and, 44
Host, susceptible, 136–137
Household contact, disease transmission and, 27
HRIG (Human rabies immune globin), 92
Human diploid cell vaccine (HDCV), 92
Human rabies immune globin (HRIG), 92
Humoral immunity, 45

I

IgA (Immunoglobulin A), defined, 43
IgD (Immunoglobulin D), defined, 44
IgE (Immunoglobulin E), defined, 44
IgG (Immunoglobulin G), defined, 44
Immune response, 38–45
    Immunoglobulin M (IgM) and, 44
Immune system, 33–41
    anatomy of, **35**
    cells of, **41**
    function of, 37–38
    structure of, 35–37
Immunity
    acquired, 42
    active, 43
    antibody-mediated, 45
    cell-mediated, 45
    humoral, 45

inherited, 42
nonspecific, 38, 39
passive, 43
specific, defined, 38
Immunizations
    recommended, **129**
    *see also* specific disease
Immunoglobulin A (IgA), defined, 43
Immunoglobulin D (IgD), defined, 44
Immunoglobulin E (IgE), defined, 44
Immunoglobulin G (IgG), defined, 44
Immunoglobulin M (IgM), defined, 44
Incubation period
    defined, 28, **29**
    *see also* specific disease
Indirect exposure, 24
Infection
    chain of, **27**, 135–137
    signs of, **40**
Infection control
    history of modern, 2–3
    introduced, 1–7
    OSHA and, 10–12
Infectious disease
    causes of, **25**
    versus communicable disease, **24**
    defined, 23
    stages of, **29**
Inflammatory response, 40–42
Influenza, overview of, 75–76
Inherited immunity, defined, 42
In-hospital isolation, 120–122
Injuries, phlebotomy (blood-drawing), 115
Integumentary system, nonspecific immunity and, 39
Interferon, 42
Isolation
    in-hospital, 120–122
    out-of-hospital, 123
Isoniazid, tuberculosis and, 106
IV connector injuries, 115

Kaposi's sarcoma, **53**
Killer T cells, 45

*Klebsiella pneumoniae*, 89
Koplik's spots, 83

Latent period, defined, **29**
Laundering, communicable disease and, 126
Left ventricular block, 81
Legal issues
    ADA and, 14
    Needlestick Prevention and Safety Act of 2000 and, 14–15
    OSHA and, 10–12
    Ryan White Care Act and, 12–14
*Legionella*, 89
Legionella pneumophila, 76–77
Legionellosis, overview of, 76–77
Leukocytes
    immune system and, 37
    inflammatory response and, 40
Lice, overview of, 77–79
Lindane, scabies and, 99
Lingual tonsils, 35
Lister, Joseph, germ theory and, 3
Listeria monocytogenes, 79
Listeriosis, overview of, 79–80
Lupus, 38
Lyme disease, overview of, 81–82
Lymph nodes, defined, 36
Lymphatic vessels, defined, 36
Lymphocytes, 36
Lymphotoxin, 45
Lysozyme, nonspecific immunity and, 39
*Lyssavirus*, 91–93

Macrophages
    inflammatory response and, 40
    phagocytosis and, 41–42
Malaria, 25
    vector borne transmission of disease and, 26
Mantoux test, 106
Masks, communicable disease and, 124, **125**
Mast cells, Immunoglobulin E (IgE) and, 44
Material Safety Data Sheets (MSDS), defined, 116

Measles, overview of, 82–83
Medical devices
    with built-in safety features, **115**
    communicable disease and, 114–5
Meningitis, Lyme disease and, 81
Meningococcal meningitis, overview of, 84–85
Method of travel, defined, 137
Minocycline, meningococcal meningitis and, 84
Monocytes, 36
Mononucleosis, overview of, 85–86
*Moraxella catarrhalis*, 89
*Morbilli*, 82
MSDS (Material Safety Data Sheets), 116
Multiple sclerosis, 38
Mumps, overview of, 86–87
Myasthenia gravis, **38**
*mycobacterium tuberculosis*, **105**
*Mycoplasma pneumoniae*, 89
Myocarditis, 81

National Clinician's Post-Exposure Prophylaxis Hotline (PEPline), **144**
National Fire Protection Association (NFPA), infection control and, 16
Natural killer cells, 42
Needles
    handling/using, 118
    one-handed recap technique, **120**
Needlestick Prevention and Safety Act of 2000, 14–15
Negligence, defined, 16–17
*Neisseria gonorrhea*, 65
*Neisseria meningitidis*, 84
Neonates, Immunoglobulin G (IgG) and, 44
Neutrophils
    inflammatory response and, 40
    phagocytosis and, 41–42
NFA (National Fire Academy), infection control and, 16
NFPA (National Fire Protection Association), infection control and, 16
Nonspecific immunity, 39, 42
    defined, 38
Nonsteroidal anti-inflammatory drugs (NSAIDS), mononucleosis and, 85
Nosocomial infections, isolation and, 120
Notification by request, Ryan White care act and, 14
NSAIDS (Nonsteroidal anti-inflammatory drugs), mononucleosis and, 85
Nuchal rigidity, meningococcal meningitis and, 84

Occupational exposure to bloodborne pathogens rule, established by OSHA, 10–12
Occupational Safety and Health Administration (OSHA) *See* OSHA
Oocyst, 60
OPIM (Other potentially infectious material), defined, 28
OSHA
    200 log, 145
    300 log, 145
    approved plans, **11**
    occupational exposure to bloodborne pathogens rule established, 10–12
    post exposure reporting requirements, 145
    sharps container regulation, 113–114
Other potentially infectious material (OPIM), defined, 28
Out-of-hospital isolation, 123

Palatine tonsils, 35
Paramyxovirus, 86
Passive immunity, defined, 43
Pasteur, Louis, germ theory and, 2
Patient management *See* specific disease
Pediculicide, 78–79
Pediculosis humanus capitis, 77
Pediculosis humanus corporis, 77
Pediculosis, overview of, 77–79
Pelvic inflammatory disease (PID), gonorrhea and, 65
Penicillin, syphilis and, 103
PEPline (National Clinician's Post-Exposure Prophylaxis Hotline), **144**
Percutaneous injuries, estimation of number of, 14–15
Peripheral neuropathy, Lyme disease and, 81
Permethrin, scabies and, 99
Personal health, 17–18, 128–131
    physical exams and, 128
    vaccinations and, 128–30
Personal protective equipment (PPE), 123–127
Perspiration, nonspecific immunity and, 39
Pertussis, overview of, 87–89
Petechial rash, meningococcal meningitis and, 84
Peyer's patches, 37
Phagocytosis, 36, 41–42
    inflammatory response and, 40

Pharyngeal tonsils, 35
Phlebotomy (blood-drawing) injuries, 115
Physical exams, personal health and, 128
PID (Pelvic inflammatory disease), gonorrhea and, 65
Pinworms, 25
Placenta, Immunoglobulin G (IgG) and, 44
Pneumonia, overview of, 89–91
Portal of entry, 136
    defined, 137
Portal of exit, defined, 136
Post exposure, 141–149
    counseling, 148
    education, 148
    first aid, 142
    OSHA reporting requirements, 145
    physical strategies, 148–149
    reporting, 142, 144
    return to work, 146
    stress management, 146–149
    testing, 145
        and follow up, 144
PPE (Personal protective equipment), 123–127
Prostatitis, gonorrhea and, 65
Protective equipment, personal, 123–127
Protective measures *See* specific disease
Protozoans, defined, 25
Proximate cause, described, 17
Psoriasis, **38**
Pthirus pubis, 77
Purulent urinary discharges, Chlamydia and, 58
Pyrazinamide, tuberculosis and, 106
Pythiriasis, overview of, 77–79

Questions, test review, 151–157

Rabies, overview of, 91–93
Recombivax HB, 69–70
Reporting, post exposure, 142, 144
Reservoir of infection, defined, 136
Respirators, communicable disease and, 124
Respiratory system, nonspecific immunity and, 39

Return to work, authorization, 131
Return to work authorization, post exposure, 146
Rheumatic fever, 38
Rheumatoid arthritis, **38**
Ribavirin, 67
*Rickettsia rickettsii*, Rocky Mountain Spotted Fever and, 94
Rickettsias, defined, 25
Rifampin
     meningococcal meningitis and, 84
     tuberculosis and, 106
Ringworm, 25
Rocky Mountain Spotted Fever, 25
     overview of, 93–94
     vector borne transmission of disease and, 26
Routes of transmission *See* specific disease
Routine notification, Ryan White care act and, 14
Rubella, overview of, 94–97
Rubella, rash, **96**
Rubeola, overview of, 82–83
RVA (Adsorbed vaccine), 92
Ryan White Comprehensive AIDS Resources Emergency (CARE) Act of
     1990, 12–14

Safe work practices
     communicable disease and, 116–122
     examples of, **117**
*Salmonella*, 97
Salmonellosis, overview of, 97–98
Scabies, overview of, 98–100
Scalpels, handling/using, 118
Scleroderma, **38**
Sebum, nonspecific immunity and, 39
Semmelweis, Ignaz, 2
Septic arthritis, 66
Seroconversion, 27–30
     defined, 28
     progression, **28**
Sexual transmission of disease, 26
Sexually transmitted diseases (STDs), 26
Sharps containers, communicable disease and, 113–114
Sharps, handling/using, 118–120
*Shigella*, 100
Shigellosis, overview of, 100–101

Signs/symptoms *See* specific disease
Skin, immune system and, 37
Sleeping sickness, 25
Source of infection, defined, 136
Specific immunity
    components of, 43–44
    defined, 38
    described, 42–45
Spiramycin, meningococcal meningitis and, 84
Spleen, defined, 36
*Sarcoptes scabiei*, 98
Standard precautions, **121**
    defined, 120
*Staphylococcus aureus*, 89
*Streptococcus pneumoniae*, 89
Streptomycin, tuberculosis and, 106
Stress
    managing, post exposure, 146–149
    physical/emotional signs of, **147**
Susceptible
    defined, 51
    *see also* specific disease
Susceptible host, defined, 136–137
Sutures, handling/using, 118
Syphilis, 26
    overview of, 101–103
Systemic bacteremia, 66

T cells, 45
T lymphocytes, 45
    defined, 36
T suppressor cells, 45
Tapeworms, 25
TB (Tuberculosis), 4
    airborne transmission, 26
Test review questions, 151–157
Testing, post exposure, 145
Tetanus
    jaw contractions of, **104**
    overview of, 103–105
    prophylaxis, 92
    toxoid, 105
Tetanus immune globulin (TIG), 104

Tetracycline, Rocky Mountain Spotted Fever, 93
Thrombocytopenia, rubella and, 95
Thymus, defined, 36
TIG (Tetanus immune globulin), 104
Tinea, 25
Tonsils
    lingual, 35
    palatine, 35
    pharyngeal, 35
Transmission mode, defined, 136
Transmission-based precautions, defined, 120–121
*Treponema pallidum* bacteria, 101
Tuberculosis (TB), 4
    airborne transmission, 26
    overview of, 105–106
Tumors, immune system and, 37
Typhus, 25

Uniforms, communicable disease and, 126
Urethral strictures, gonorrhea and, 65

Vaccinations, personal health and, 128–30
Vacomycin, pneumonia and, 90
Varicella-zoster virus, 58
Vector borne transmission of disease, 26
Vermiform appendix, 36–37
Viruses, defined, 24

White blood cells, inflammatory response and, 40
White, Ryan, biography of, **13**
Whooping cough, overview of, 87–89
Window phase, defined, 28, **29**
Woolsorters' disease, overview of, 55–56

Zovirax, 73
    herpes simplex and, 74